T0264002

Complementary and Alternative Medicine, Part II: Herbal Supplements and Vitamins

Editor

STEPHEN D. KRAU

NURSING CLINICS
OF NORTH AMERICA

www.nursing.theclinics.com

Consulting Editor
STEPHEN D. KRAU

March 2021 • Volume 56 • Number 1

ELSEVIER

1600 John F. Kennedy Boulevard • Suite 1800 • Philadelphia, Pennsylvania, 19103-2899

http://www.theclinics.com

NURSING CLINICS OF NORTH AMERICA Volume 56, Number 1
March 2021 ISSN 0029-6465, ISBN-13: 978-0-323-76117-8

Editor: Kerry Holland
Developmental Editor: Axell Ivan Jade M. Purificacion

© **2021 Elsevier Inc. All rights reserved.**

This periodical and the individual contributions contained in it are protected under copyright by Elsevier, and the following terms and conditions apply to their use:

Photocopying
Single photocopies of single articles may be made for personal use as allowed by national copyright laws. Permission of the Publisher and payment of a fee is required for all other photocopying, including multiple or systematic copying, copying for advertising or promotional purposes, resale, and all forms of document delivery. Special rates are available for educational institutions that wish to make photocopies for non-profit educational classroom use. For information on how to seek permission visit www.elsevier.com/permissions or call: (+44) 1865 843830 (UK)/ (+1) 215 239 3804 (USA).

Derivative Works
Subscribers may reproduce tables of contents or prepare lists of articles including abstracts for internal circulation within their institutions. Permission of the Publisher is required for resale or distribution outside the institution. Permission of the Publisher is required for all other derivative works, including compilations and translations (please consult www.elsevier.com/permissions).

Electronic Storage or Usage
Permission of the Publisher is required to store or use electronically any material contained in this periodical, including any article or part of an article (please consult www.elsevier.com/permissions). Except as outlined above, no part of this publication may be reproduced, stored in a retrieval system or transmitted in any form or by any means, electronic, mechanical, photocopying, recording or otherwise, without prior written permission of the Publisher.

Notice
No responsibility is assumed by the Publisher for any injury and/or damage to persons or property as a matter of products liability, negligence or otherwise, or from any use or operation of any methods, products, instructions or ideas contained in the material herein. Because of rapid advances in the medical sciences, in particular, independent verification of diagnoses and drug dosages should be made.

Although all advertising material is expected to conform to ethical (medical) standards, inclusion in this publication does not constitute a guarantee or endorsement of the quality or value of such product or of the claims made of it by its manufacturer.

Nursing Clinics of North America (ISSN 0029-6465) is published quarterly by Elsevier Inc., 360 Park Avenue South, New York, NY 10010-1710. Months of issue are March, June, September, and December. Periodicals postage paid at New York, NY and additional mailing offices. Subscription price per year is, $163.00 (US individuals), $669.00 (US institutions), $275.00 (international individuals), $692.00 (international institutions), $231.00 (Canadian individuals), $692.00 (Canadian institutions), $100.00 (US and Canadian students), and $135.00 (international students). To receive student/resident rate, orders must be accompanied by name of affiliated institution, date of term, and the signature of program/residency coordinator on institution letterhead. Orders will be billed at individual rate until proof of status is received. Foreign air speed delivery is included in all *Clinics* subscription prices. All prices are subject to change without notice. **POSTMASTER:** Send address changes to *Nursing Clinics,* Elsevier Health Sciences Division, Subscription Customer Service, 3251 Riverport Lane, Maryland Heights, MO 63043. **Customer Service: Telephone: 1-800-654-2452** (U.S. and Canada); **1-314-447-8871 (outside U.S. and Canada). Fax: 1-314-447-8029. E-mail: journalscustomerservice-usa@ elsevier.com** (for print support) and **journalsonlinesupport-usa@elsevier.com** (for online support).

Nursing Clinics of North America is covered in *EMBASE/Excerpta Medica, MEDLINE/PubMed (Index Medicus), Social Sciences Citation Index, Current Contents, ASCA, Cumulative Index to Nursing, RNdex Top 100,* and Allied Health Literature and International Nursing Index (INI).

Contributors

CONSULTING EDITOR

STEPHEN D. KRAU, PhD, RN, CNE
Associate Professor (Ret), Vanderbilt University School of Nursing, Nashville, Tennessee, USA

EDITOR

STEPHEN D. KRAU, PhD, RN, CNE
Associate Professor (Ret), Vanderbilt University School of Nursing, Nashville, Tennessee, USA

AUTHORS

LINDA K. DARNELL, MSN, RN
Associate Professor, School of Nursing, Austin Peay State University, Clarksville, Tennessee, USA

DEBORAH L. ELLISON, PhD, MSN, BSN
Professor of Nursing, Austin Peay State University, School of Nursing, Clarksville, Tennessee, USA

AMANDA J. FLAGG, PhD, RN, MSN/EdM, ACNS, CNE
Associate Professor, Middle Tennessee State University (MTSU) School of Nursing, Murfreesboro, Tennessee, USA

SHONDELL V. HICKSON, DNP, MSN, APRN, ACNS-BC, FNP-BC
Professor, School of Nursing, Austin Peay State University, Clarksville, Tennessee, USA

CHERYL B. HINES, EdD, MSN, CRNA
Clinical Assistant Professor, Capstone College of Nursing, The University of Alabama Tuscaloosa, Tuscaloosa, Alabama, USA

AMY S.D. LEE, DNP, ARNP, WHNP-BC
Clinical Associate Professor, Capstone College of Nursing, The University of Alabama, Tuscaloosa, Alabama, USA

LEIGH ANN McINNIS, PhD, FNP-BC, RN
Professor, Nursing, Middle Tennessee State University, Murfreesboro, Tennessee, USA

HEATHER R. MORAN, MSN, BSN, CRRN, CMSRN
Assistant Professor of Nursing, Austin Peay State University, School of Nursing, Clarksville, Tennessee, USA

ANGELA MOREHEAD, DNP, FNP-BC, RN
Assistant Professor, Nursing, Middle Tennessee State University, Murfreesboro, Tennessee, USA

MARCIA A. PUGH, DNP, MSN, MBA, HCM, RN
CEO, Greene County Health System, Eutaw, Alabama, USA

MARIA A. REVELL, PhD, MSN, RN, COI
Executive Director, Tennessee State University, School of Nursing, Nashville, Tennessee, USA

SHANNON L. SMITH-STEPHENS, DNP, APRN-BC, SANE
Assistant Professor of Nursing, Morehead State University, Morehead, Kentucky, USA; Contract Medical Provider, Department of Juvenile Justice, Owner/Provider, Shannon L. Smith-Stephens, DNP, APRN-BC, PLLC, Olive Hill, Kentucky, USA

SHERRI L. STEVENS, PhD, RN
Associate Professor, School of Nursing, Middle Tennessee State University, Murfreesboro, Tennessee, USA

SHERIN F. TAHMASBI, DNP, FNP-C
Associate Professor, Tennessee State University, School of Nursing, Nashville, Tennessee, USA

NATASHA TAHMASEBI, BSc
Medical Student, Kings College University, London, England

DANIELLE WHITE, MSN, RN
Associate Professor, School of Nursing, Austin Peay State University, Clarksville, Tennessee, USA

CHRISTOPHER TY WILLIAMS, DNP, RN, ACNP-BC, FNP-BC, CNE
Assistant Professor, School of Nursing, Vanderbilt University, Nashville, Tennessee, USA

Contents

The Food and Drug Administration (FDA) classifies herbal preparations as food supplements. New herbal supplements and products are not governed by the strict FDA drug approval process and there is no premarket approval required. The FDA prohibits manufacturers and distributors from marketing adulterated or misbranded products but does not rigorously define safe practices. Scientific evidence related to herbal supplements is limited. Herbal supplements have been associated with adverse reactions and herbal-drug interactions. Information and precautions for 20 common herbal supplements, including St. John's wort, ginseng, echinacea, and ginkgo, are reviewed. Resources for consumers and health care professionals are highlighted.

Vitamin B6, a cofactor in many biochemical reactions in the cells of living organisms, is an essential coenzyme for various catabolic and anabolic processes. Although vitamin B6 deficiency in young healthy women with a balanced diet is thought to be unusual, it can be seen with certain medications, health conditions, and dietary deficits, as well as aging. Vitamin B6 deficiency is associated with a variety of ill health effects, and correction of deficiency is considered beneficial. Women particularly are affected by unique health issues that are part of the array of disorders potentially alleviated through vitamin B6 supplementation.

The fat-soluble vitamins are vitamins A, D, E, and K. Each vitamin has unique characteristics and contributes to the overall health of an individual. These vitamins have complex absorption, metabolism, and distribution elements that provide protection to the cells in the body as well as many organs. Fat-soluble vitamins, once ingested and processed, are stored in the body for use. Most fat-soluble vitamins are obtained from fruits, vegetables, nuts, and animals.

Vitamin D can be obtained from diet, direct sunlight, or supplementation. The most common form is synthesized in the skin after exposure to ultraviolet B radiation. Nevertheless, the thought is that vitamin D is more of a multifunctional hormone or prohormone. This is because vitamin D plays contributes to many processes in the body. Calcitriol has been shown to have enhancing effects on the immune system, the cardiovascular system, the endocrine system, and other metabolic pathways. There is evidence that vitamin D has also a role in depression, pain, and cancer.

Herbal medicine is the art and science of using herbs, for health promotion and preventing and treating illnesses that are not usually considered part of standard medical care. It is the leading therapy among complementary and alternative medicine (CAM) use in the United States. Using herbal supplements to improve or stave off the effects of normal cognitive aging is appealing to many patients because of the misconception that "natural" therapies have no adverse effects. Herbal supplement manufacturers often saturate consumers with direct advertisement on various media platforms with alternative treatment of a variety of ailments.

The use of alternative therapies for health problems specific to women is increasing. As many as 67% of women admit to using complementary therapies of some kind, including supplements, chiropractic intervention, acupuncture, and acupressure. Many women turn to herbal supplements because they think that pharmacologic interventions are unsafe or not effective. Current literature provides conflicting information regarding many complementary and alternative therapies, including herbal supplements. Although most are not harmful, it is important to review the safety and efficacy of supplements for women's health issues.

Viral infections and their emergence continue to pose a threat to human lives. Up to the present, there are limited numbers of vaccines that effectively work and few antivirals licensed for use in clinical practice. Added to this is the increase in antiviral resistance, meaning that drugs that do work are at risk of reduced efficacy. The recent global pandemic of coronavirus 2019 has provided evidence for the risk of a preventative vaccination and effective treatment of viruses' subsequent consequences. The aim of this article is to review traditional and herbal treatments for infections, specifically addressing gastrointestinal and respiratory viral infections.

Fever is a natural body defense and a common symptom of disease. Herbs have been used for thousands of years to treat fever. Many herbs have anti-inflammatory properties. Some are useful in reducing the release of cytokines and mediators of inflammation, whereas others work as natural aspirins to inhibit cyclooxygenase. In addition, herbs have known antipathogenic properties and can be effective in the treatment of infection from numerous microorganisms. Last, in traditional Chinese medicine, herbs are used to restore imbalances between the nonpathogenic and the pathogenic clearing interior heat and treating heat patterns in a variety of ways.

Garlic originated in West China and has been used for its health qualities since 2600 BCE. Garlic was brought to Great Britain in 1548 from the Mediterranean Sea. Early uses of garlic were to treat gastric infections, fevers, and diarrhea. Fresh garlic has the most health benefits through the compound allicin. Health benefits of garlic include the prevention and treatment of cardiovascular disease, antioxidant effects, antimicrobial effects, and reduction of cancer risks.

NURSING CLINICS OF NORTH AMERICA

SERIES OF RELATED INTEREST

Critical Care Nursing Clinics of North America
https://www.ccnursing.theclinics.com/
Advances in Family Practice Nursing
http://www.advancesinfamilypracticenursing.com/

THE CLINICS ARE AVAILABLE ONLINE!
Access your subscription at:
www.theclinics.com

Preface

Complementary and Alternative Medications: A Growing Phenomenon

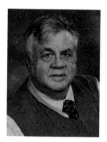

Stephen D. Krau, PhD, RN, CNE
Editor

The link between natural herbs and medications and formally approved medications is historically undeniable. For example, the foxglove plant was used for centuries to treat cardiac conditions before it was processed and served as the basis for prescription digitoxin medications. During the US Civil War, the bark of weeping willow trees was used as a pain reliever before science identified it contained acetylsalicylic acid, more commonly known as aspirin. Currently, over 40 billion dollars of noninsurance reimbursed dollars are spent on complementary or alternative medications (CAMs) in the United States annually. It is almost impossible to view a mainstream channel television program without seeing a commercial for an alternative medication to improve memory, reduce pain, or assist in weight loss. Even on news channels there have been physicians advocating for the over-the-counter use of vitamin D and zinc to ameliorate the impact of COVID-19 on individuals. In industrialized countries, it is estimated by the World Health Organization that 30% to 80% of adults use some form of CAM to prevent or treat illnesses, including over 60 million in the United States.[1] The variant medications and claims increase in numbers annually. These medications are not "approved" by the Food and Drug Administration in the same manner as medications that can only be obtained with a prescription. In 1992, however, the US Congress established the Office of Alternative Medicine, which is now called "The National Center for Complementary and Alternative Health (NCCAM) at the National Institutes of Health."[2] NCCAM defines CAM as a group of diverse medical and health care systems, practices, and products that are not presently considered to be part of 'conventional medicine' and integrative medicine as the art of [combining] mainstream medical therapies for which there is some high quality scientific evidence of safety and effectiveness. This differs from "Holistic Medicine," which is considered an

Nurs Clin N Am 56 (2021) xi–xii
https://doi.org/10.1016/j.cnur.2020.11.001
0029-6465/21/© 2020 Published by Elsevier Inc.

approach to medical care that emphasizes the study of all aspects of a person's health, including physical, psychological, spiritual, social, economic and cultural factors.[2] The previous issue of *Nursing Clinics of North America* (December 2020) focused on nonmedicine therapeutic interventions of CAM. This issue focuses on medicines that fall into the CAM categories. This issue is by no means a complete inventory of CAM medications but presents and overviews of many common medications, their uses, and some of the precautions that should be considered when using CAM medications.

The probability that a patient is taking at least one CAM medication is 30% to 80%.[2] In addition, due to the characteristics of the majority of people who take CAM medications, this patient is white, between 25 and 49 years old, with some college education, and an income above $35,000 annually.[2] More than likely, only about 20% of the physicians who care for these patients is aware their patients are taking CAM medications. It is important that any ingestible therapies be ascertained on initial patient intake, as many patients believe if a substance is accessible over the counter, or does not require a medical prescription, that the substance is not a medication. Many of these substances can interact with medications that are prescribed, which can have an adverse interaction effect.

Expect to see a tremendous growth in CAM medications in the next few years. In addition, pharmacists, nurses, and physicians are aware that these modalities are quickly becoming mainstream. As a result of the market, use, and growth, information about CAMs is gradually being incorporated into health care professional curricula.

Stephen D. Krau, PhD, RN, CNE
Vanderbilt University School of Nursing
21st Avenue South
Nashville, TN 37240, USA

E-mail address:
sdkrau@outlook.com

REFERENCES

1. Alternative medicine. Expanding medical horizons. A report to the National Institute of Health on alternative medical systems and practices in the United States. Chantilly (VA): U.S. Government Printing Office.
2. Rosenbaum CC. The history of complementary and alternative medicine in the U.S. Ann Pharmacother 2007;41:1256–60.

Herbal Supplements
Precautions and Safe Use

Christopher Ty Williams, DNP, RN, ACNP-BC, FNP-BC, CNE

KEYWORDS

- Herbal supplements • Herbal medicine • Botanicals • Precautions
- Herbal-drug interactions • Safe use

KEY POINTS

- Scientific evidence related to herbal dietary supplements is limited.
- The FDA does not approve herbal dietary supplements before market, as they do with new drugs.
- Herbal dietary supplements can cause significant adverse effects and herbal-drug interactions.
- Resources are available for consumers and health care professionals to stay up to date with herbal dietary supplements.

INTRODUCTION

Federal law defines an herbal supplement, also known as a botanical, herbal remedy, or herbal dietary supplement, as a type of dietary supplement containing one or more herb, plant (other than tobacco), algae, fungi, or lichen that is often used in addition to traditional medical treatments to preserve or recover health.[1–4] Sales of herbal products in the United States reached $6 billion in 2013 and exceeded $8 billion in 2018.[5] The US Food and Drug Administration (FDA) classifies herbal remedies, medications, and supplements as food supplements and applies different regulatory standards than those governing conventional foods and drugs.[1,6] As such, herbal supplements are not affected by pharmaceutical legislation.[1,7] Furthermore, new herbal supplements do not receive premarket approval and are not subject to the strict FDA drug approval process, five steps that include discovery, preclinical research, clinical research, review, and postmarket safety monitoring.[8]

Although only providing limited regulation, the FDA does prohibit herbal supplement manufacturers and distributors from marketing products that are adulterated or misbranded.[9] The FDA is responsible for investigating and acting on violations once

Funding: None.
Disclaimer: The author declares no conflict of interest.
School of Nursing, Vanderbilt University, 461 21st Avenue South, Nashville, TN 37240, USA
E-mail address: christopher.t.williams@vanderbilt.edu

Nurs Clin N Am 56 (2021) 1–21
https://doi.org/10.1016/j.cnur.2020.10.001
0029-6465/21/© 2020 Elsevier Inc. All rights reserved.

nursing.theclinics.com

they have reached the marketplace.[1,9] Approximately half of FDA class 1 drug recalls since 2004 were related to the adulteration of dietary supplements with banned ingredients.[10] It has also been reported that dietary supplements remain on store shelves even after FDA has issued recalls.[11,12]

Manufacturers themselves are responsible for ensuring product safety and accurate labeling.[2] Because there is no incentive for conducting large, diverse, randomized controlled trials that explore safety, efficacy, and risk, scientific evidence is scarce.[10,13] Because the FDA does not regulate the purity of herbal supplements, formulae, potency, or actions, adverse reactions and toxicities vary within and between manufacturers.[13,14]

Frequently used herbal supplements, including echinacea, garlic, ginkgo, and St. John's wort, can produce mild to severe adverse reactions and lead to clinically significant herbal-drug interactions.[15,16] However, little scientific evidence is available to describe the safety, risks, and efficacy of these herbal supplements.[15,17] This article provides baseline knowledge about the regulation of herbal supplements, discusses common herbal-drug interactions, identifies safety implications for individuals and special groups, describes 20 herbal supplements and important precautions, and highlights resources for health care providers and consumers.

BACKGROUND

The World Health Organization has defined herbal medicines similarly to the FDA, as labeled products that contain an active ingredient and any part of the plant, above or below ground, or plant material.[17] Herbal supplements come in a variety of forms and are consumed as pills, tinctures, teas, applied topically, or added to bath water.[6] Herbal remedies have been used for thousands of years; today, herbal supplements are commonly thought to enhance health, promote wellness and a sense of well-being, boost immunity, and minimize symptoms of chronic diseases, including anxiety, cancer, chronic pain, fatigue, and memory loss.[1,11,14,18,19] Worldwide, an estimated 80% of the population relies on herbal medicines as a standard of care.[10] In a 2015 US survey of 26,157 consumers related to views and perceptions of medications and pharmacy, 35% reported using at least one herbal medication or supplement, with an average of 2.6 supplements used per consumer.[19,20]

Unlike China, Germany, and Japan, the United States does not strictly regulate dietary supplements.[17] Federal oversight is provided via the Dietary Supplement Health Education Act (DSHEA) of 1994.[9,21] The DSHEA solidified the definition of dietary supplements and grouped them separately from drugs. Under the DSHEA, dietary supplements are required to contain the following language: "this product is not intended to diagnose, treat, cure, or prevent disease." When producing a new herbal supplement or herbal product, drug developers and manufacturers are expected to notify the FDA; however, they are not required to complete a new drug application.[7,11] The FDA implemented new rules in 2007 that mandated Good Manufacturing Practices (GMPs), which include proper, accurate labeling; a product free of adulterants; and establishment of standards for manufacturing equipment and personnel.[22] Despite these standards, associating adverse reactions with specific plants remains problematic, because frequently supplements contain multiple unregulated compounds.[13] In 2013, it was reported that over a 3-year period, FDA GMP inspectors cited 70% of dietary supplement producers. In response, organizations including the Academy of Medicine and Center for Science in the Public Interest have called for reform of the DSHEA.[22]

SAFETY

Because herbal supplements are not regulated by the FDA, clinicians do not have access to evidence-based drug monographs or prescribing guidelines. Although drug databases and electronic medical records frequently include herbal supplement content, the information posted has not been validated by the FDA. To combat this, consumers and health care providers must be aware of common precautions to prevent adverse reaction and herbal-drug interactions. Consumers should consult health care providers on planned use, educate themselves about the supplement, follow instructions on labels, and monitor for adverse reactions.[6,13,15]

Health care providers play important roles in promoting the informed, safe use of herbal supplements and preventing or identifying adverse reactions and herbal-drug interactions. The importance of documenting a thorough medical history and providing appropriate patient education cannot be overstated.[3,6,15] In the 2012 National Health Interview Survey study, investigators studied the disclosure of complementary and alternative medicines in primary care and found that only approximately 75% of those who admitted using herbal supplements disclosed their use to their health care provider.[23] Reasons for not disclosing included not being specifically asked about complementary and alternative medicine and not believing the health care provider needed to know, highlighting the importance of providers asking targeted, specific questions during a patient interview.[13,23] To combat this lack of disclosure, patients should be asked about herbal supplements when medications are reviewed at every visit.[24] Providers should use multiple specific terminologies related to dietary supplements and encourage patients to bring the containers of any supplements for review.[25] Providers should record supplement use in the medical record and develop patient-specific teaching about the drug, herbal supplement, adverse reactions, and potential interactions.[1,2]

Related to the lack of federal oversight on the production of herbal supplements, GMPs cannot be monitored or guaranteed. As written, GMPs provide flexible quality criteria for manufacturers, which can lead to variability in efficacy and safety.[22,26] Furthermore, the exact plant species, parts of the plant used, harvesting, storage, processing protocols, formula standardizations, accuracy of labeling, purity and adulteration, and efficacy are neither well described nor regulated.

Special attention should be paid to vulnerable populations and their use of herbal supplements. One such population is elderly patients, who frequently take multiple prescription and over-the-counter medications, resulting in an increased risk of adverse effects and drug interactions. In a systematic review of herbal medication use among elderly adults, use was described as common, underscoring the need to focus special attention on this population.[27] For women who are pregnant or breastfeeding, no regulatory guidelines exist to protect this population and use of herbal supplements is generally not recommended.[28] Similarly, there is no evidence to support the safe use of herbal supplements in children.

HERB-DRUG INTERACTIONS

Associated with the increased use of herbal supplements is an increase in the potential for adverse reactions, including herbal-drug interactions. Well-documented examples of adverse effects related to herbal supplements are found in case studies and clinical trials.[15,29] However, available data are not representative of the general population. Clinically relevant herbal-drug interactions most commonly present as pharmacokinetic interactions related to the movement of the drug through the body, including disruptions in drug absorption, distribution, metabolism, and excretion.[15,24,29] Competition for resources may lead to variable concentrations of a drug, particularly with frequent metabolizers including the liver's cytochrome P-450 isoenzymes CYP3A4, CYP1A2, CYP2C9, and CYP2D6.[15,24] Pharmacodynamic interactions are related to the body's biologic response to drug reactions and occur less commonly.[15,24] They can occur when an herbal supplement amplifies or antagonizes the clinical effects of a drug without increasing the drug's serum concentration.[10,15]

Evidence describing herbal-drug interactions is limited and can be discussed in terms of risks associated with concurrent use of specific classes of drugs. **Table 1** highlights potential herbal-drug interactions, including the effect of the interaction on a medication's effectiveness and risk profile.

Anticoagulants, particularly warfarin, have been reported to interact with garlic, American ginseng, milk thistle, and St. John's wort, resulting in reduced medication serum levels and reduced medication activity.[10,24] Conversely, gingko has been associated with increased serum warfarin levels and increased medication activity. Patients taking warfarin should be educated about therapeutic serum drug levels, the international normalized ratio, and potential interactions with herbal supplements. Patients who choose to take herbal supplements concurrently should be followed closely.[10,24]

Cardiovascular medications, including antihypertensives, digoxin, and statins, have been shown to interact with multiple herbal supplements.[10,24] St. John's wort, frequently used in association with mood disorders and mild to moderate depression, is associated with reduced effectiveness of the calcium-channel blocker verapamil, digoxin, and statins.[10,24] American ginseng has been shown to interact with antihypertensive drugs, leading to an increase in medication effectiveness. Green tea extract has been associated with reduced activity of β-blockers, and milk thistle with reduced activity of losartan.[30]

Little is known about herbal-drug interactions associated with diabetes drugs. However, certain herbal supplements have been associated with unpredictable effects on serum glucose.[24,26] For instance, devil's claw and figwort are associated with hyperglycemia, whereas alfalfa, celery, eucalyptus, garlic, ginger, Asian ginseng, juniper, nettle, psyllium, and sage have been associated with hypoglycemia. Asian ginseng has been associated with a possibly additive effect in patients taking oral antidiabetic medications and insulin.[24,26]

Herbal supplements metabolized by the same pathway as human immunodeficiency virus/AIDS drugs, namely St. John's wort, may lead to decreased serum levels of antiretrovirals and should be closely monitored.[13,16,24] Bulk laxatives, including psyllium, made from the husks of the *Plantago ovata* plant's seeds, have been associated with decreased serum drug levels, particularly carbamazepine and lithium.[24] Herbal ingredients known to be hormonally active include alfalfa, aniseed, bayberry, black cohosh, American and Asian ginseng, horseradish, motherwort, pleurisy root, red clover, saw palmetto, vervain, and wild carrot.[26]

TWENTY COMMON HERBAL SUPPLEMENTS

In the following sections and in **Table 2**, 20 commonly used herbal supplements are described, including reported uses, adverse effects, and precautions. When available, Alternative Medicine Effectiveness Rating Definitions, developed by Natural Medicines' Therapeutic Research Center, are provided.[31] Definitions are evidence-based and standardized, and include the following ratings: effective, likely effective, possibly effective, possibly ineffective, likely ineffective, and ineffective.[31]

Table 1
Potential drug interactions of common herbal supplements

Herbal Supplement	Drugs or Drug Classes	Interaction
Black cohosh *Actaea racemosa*	Amiodarone, fexofenadine, glyburide, statins	Reduced medication effectiveness
Echinacea *Echinacea purpurea*	Antipsychotics, antidepressants, oral contraceptives	Reduced medication effectiveness
Garlic *Allium sativum*	Oral contraceptives, HIV/AIDS drugs, immunosuppressants, antituberculosis drugs, drugs transported by P-glycoprotein, including colchicine, digoxin, doxorubicin, quinidine, rosuvastatin, tacrolimus, prograf	Reduced medication effectiveness
	Antihypertensives and anticoagulants	Increased medication effectiveness
Ginger *Zingiber officinale*	Antihypertensives (calcium channel blockers), anticoagulants, diabetes drugs	Increased medication effectiveness
	Immunosuppressants	Increased risk of adverse reactions
Ginkgo *Ginkgo biloba*	Warfarin, anticoagulants	Increased medication effectiveness
	Anxiolytics, anticonvulsants, antidepressants, diabetes drugs, HIV/AIDS drugs	Reduced medication effectiveness
Ginseng, American *Panax quinquefolius*	Warfarin, anticoagulants	Reduced medication effectiveness
	Antihypertensives, diabetes drugs	Increased medication effectiveness
Ginseng, Asian *Panax ginseng*	Calcium channel blockers, chemotherapy and HIV/AIDS drugs, certain statins and antidepressants	Reduced medication effectiveness
	Warfarin	Reduced medication effectiveness
Green tea extract *Camellia sinensis*	Anticoagulants	Increased medication effectiveness
	β-Blockers, cancer drugs, antiretrovirals	Reduced medication effectiveness
	Antipsychotics, β-adrenergic agonists, amphetamines	Increased risk of adverse reactions
Milk thistle *Silybum marianum*	Losartan, warfarin, phenytoin, diazepam	Reduced medication effectiveness
St. John's wort *Hypericum perforatum*	Cyclosporine, warfarin, protease inhibitors, irinotecan, theophylline, digoxin, venlafaxine, statins, oral contraceptives	Reduced medication effectiveness

Abbreviation: HIV, human immunodeficiency virus.
Data from Refs.[30–51]

Table 2
Twenty common herbal supplements, adverse reactions, and cautions

Herbal Supplement	Adverse Reactions	Caution
Capsicum pepper *Capsicum frutescens* or *annuum*	Anaphylaxis Abdominal pain, belching, bloating, anal burning, renal/hepatic damage Local burning, contact dermatitis, edema, erythema, flushing Rhinorrhea, lacrimation, sneezing, mucous membrane irritation	Avoid if upcoming surgery or hypersensitivity to peppers Consult provider before use with history of bleeding disorders, diabetes mellitus, or hypertension
Chamomile, German *Matricaria recutita*	Anaphylaxis, hypersensitivity reactions Confusion, drowsiness Atopic dermatitis, ecchymosis, contact dermatitis, eczema, ocular irritation	Avoid if age <2 y; pregnant; hypersensitivity to asteraceae and compositae plants, including chrysanthemums, daisies, marigolds, and ragweed Caution with asthma, hormone-sensitive conditions, or upcoming surgery
Cranberry *Vaccinium macrocarpon*	Abdominal pain, nausea, vomiting, diarrhea Nocturia, nephrolithiasis, candidiasis, vaginal pruritus Altered blood glucose	Avoid with hypersensitivity to aspirin or other salicylates Caution with asthma, atrophic gastritis, hypochlorhydria, or nephrolithiasis
Echinacea *Echinacea purpurea* and related species	Anaphylaxis, angioedema, bronchospasm, hypersensitivity reaction Abdominal pain, diarrhea, nausea, vomiting, constipation, heartburn, hepatitis Headache, dizziness, drowsiness Alteration of fertility	Avoid if history of autoimmune disorders, including multiple sclerosis, rheumatoid arthritis, or systemic lupus erythematosus Caution with atopic conditions or attempting to conceive a pregnancy
Evening primrose *Oenothera biennis*	Abdominal pain, distention, dyspepsia, flatulence, indigestion, vomiting, taste disturbance Dizziness, headache Acne, skin rash Increased risk of bleeding, decreased aggregation of platelets, decreased seizure threshold	Avoid if upcoming surgery Caution with coagulation disorders, schizophrenia, seizure disorder, pregnancy, or lactation

(continued on next page)

Table 2 *(continued)*		
Herbal Supplement	**Adverse Reactions**	**Caution**
Feverfew *Tanacetum parthenium*	Abdominal pain, nausea, vomiting, constipation, diarrhea, indigestion, flatulence, indigestion, dysgeusia, oral ulcers, gingival bleeding Anxiety, insomnia	Avoid if pregnant, age <18 y; hypersensitivity to asteraceae or compositae plants, including chrysanthemums, daisies, and marigolds
Flax/flaxseed oil *Linum usitatissimum*	Anaphylactic or hypersensitivity reactions Abdominal pain diarrhea, intestinal obstruction, nausea, vomiting Hypotension Mania	Avoid with GI disorders, obstruction, stricture, and inflammation; breast, uterine or ovarian cancer, uterine fibroids, or endometriosis; hypertriglyceridemia and open wounds Caution with bipolar disorder, bleeding disorders, diabetes mellitus, or hypothyroidism
Garlic *Allium sativum*	Anaphylaxis, angioedema, urticaria Abdominal pain, irritation, burning, belching, nausea, dyspepsia, vomiting, diarrhea, flatulence Hypotension, dizziness	Avoid with bleeding disorders; recent or upcoming surgery; or hypersensitivity to garlic or members of the liliaceae family, including lily, hyacinth, tulip, onion, leek, and chive Caution if diabetes mellitus, GI infection, peptic ulcer disease, or inflammatory bowel disease
Ginger *Zingiber officinale*	Abdominal pain, nausea, belching, distention, flatulence, diarrhea Dermatitis Hypoglycemia, CNS depression Arrhythmias	Avoid with history of gallbladder dysfunction, inflammatory bowel disease, or GI obstruction Caution with history of cardiac disease, gastric or duodenal ulcers, diabetes mellitus, HTN, hypotension, breastfeeding, or pregnancy
Ginkgo *Ginkgo biloba*	Nausea, vomiting, constipation, diarrhea, xerostomia Arrhythmias, palpitations, transient ischemic attacks, cerebrovascular accidents Edema	Avoid if attempting to conceive, are pregnant, or having surgery within 2 wk Caution if history of bleeding or seizure disorders, diabetes

(continued on next page)

Table 2 (continued)		
Herbal Supplement	Adverse Reactions	Caution
	Increased risk of bleeding, hematuria Weakness, restlessness, dizziness, drowsiness, headache Skin hypersensitivity reactions, Stevens-Johnson syndrome	mellitus, or G6PD deficiency
Ginseng, American *Panax quinquefolius*	Headache	Avoid if pregnant or having surgery within 2 wk Caution with bleeding disorders, diabetes mellitus, insomnia, hormone-sensitive conditions, ovarian or uterine cancers, uterine fibroids, endometriosis, or breast cancer
Ginseng, Asian *Panax ginseng*	Anaphylaxis, skin hypersensitivity reactions Headache, euphoria, insomnia Abdominal pain, nausea, decreased appetite, diarrhea, cholestatic hepatitis Hypertension, hypotension, tachycardia Vaginal bleeding, amenorrhea	Avoid with history of bleeding and clotting disorders, organ transplant recipients, pediatric patients, or pregnancy Caution with a history of cardiovascular disease, arrhythmias, cerebrovascular disease, autoimmune disorders, endometrial cancer or endometriosis, hormone-sensitive conditions, insomnia, or schizophrenia
Goldenseal *Hydrastis canadensis*	Abdominal pain and distention, flatulence, diarrhea, constipation, vomiting Headache, photosensitivity Skin rash Hypernatremia	Avoid with breastfeeding, pregnancy, or infants. Caution with history of bleeding disorders, diabetes mellitus, hypertension, or hypotension
Green tea *Camellia sinesis*	Nausea, vomiting, flatulence, abdominal distention, diarrhea, constipation Arrhythmias, palpitations, tachycardia, HTN Dizziness, nervousness, anxiety, restlessness, irritability, insomnia,	Avoid with breastfeeding, pregnancy, and hepatic impairment or disease. Caution with elderly patients and postmenopausal women. Caution with history of cardiovascular disease or arrhythmias, anxiety,
		(continued on next page)

Table 2
(continued)

Herbal Supplement	Adverse Reactions	Caution
	delirium Rash, urticaria Muscle spasm, seizures	diabetes mellitus, hypertension, headaches, glaucoma, psychiatric disorders, prostate cancer, renal disease, osteoporosis and gastric or duodenal ulcers
Hawthorn *Crataegus monogyna*	Nausea Dizziness, agitation, headache, insomnia Palpitations, arrhythmias, circulatory disturbance, tachycardia	Avoid if known hypersensitivity. Caution with elderly patients and concurrent cardiovascular agents, CNS depressants, and vasodilatory agents
Kava *Piper methysticum*	Hepatotoxicity, hepatic failure, hepatitis, cirrhosis Weight loss, xerostomia, mouth numbness Skin hypersensitivity reactions, scaly rash Mydriasis, oculomotor equilibrium and visual accommodation disturbances Headache, motor reflex impairment, dyskinesia	Avoid if pregnant or breast- feeding, history of or acute hepatitis, long- term ethanol use, chronic lung disease, Parkinson's disease, operating heavy machinery, or taking concurrent CNS depressants or hepatotoxic drugs. Caution in patients suffering from depressive disorders
Milk thistle *Silybum marianum*	Anaphylaxis or hypersensitivity reaction Abdominal pain, dyspepsia, nausea, vomiting, constipation, diarrhea, flatulence, laxative effect Loss of appetite, weakness Rash, pruritus, eczema, dysgeusia	Avoid with breast, ovarian, or uterine cancers, endometriosis, uterine fibroids, hormone- sensitive conditions, hypersensitivity to asteraceae or compositae plants, including chrysanthemums, daisies, or marigolds Caution in patients with diabetes mellitus
Saw palmetto *Serenoa repens*	Abdominal pain, heartburn, vomiting, dyspepsia, diarrhea, constipation, duodenal ulcer, diarrhea, constipation, hepatitis Arrhythmias, angina, heart failure, hypertension, hypotension, myocardial infarction, tachycardia, dyspnea Testicular pain, UTI, decreased libido, erectile	Avoid if breastfeeding, pregnant, or having surgery within 2 weeks Caution with bleeding disorders or hormone- sensitive conditions

(continued on next page)

Table 2
(continued)

Herbal Supplement	Adverse Reactions	Caution
	dysfunction Headache, dizziness, weakness, myalgias, insomnia Rhabdomyolysis	
St. John's wort *Hypericum perforatum*	Anorexia, nausea, vomiting, diarrhea, constipation, dyspepsia, hypoglycemia, xerostomia Agitation, dizziness, anxiety, fatigue, hypomania, irritability, lethargy, panic attack, psychosis, restlessness, serotonin-like syndrome, suicidal or homicidal ideation, vivid dreams, tremor, withdrawal symptoms Pruritus, jaundice Muscle pain, joint stiffness, Palpitations, hypertension, tachycardia, sexual dysfunction	Avoid if having difficulty conceiving a pregnancy or having surgery within 2 weeks Caution with dementia of Alzheimer's type, bipolar disorder, depression, schizophrenia, concurrent use of anesthesia, or dose greater than 2 grams per day
Valerian *Valeriana officinalis*	Agitation, excitability, fatigue, insomnia, mental dullness, morning drowsiness, restlessness, sedation, uneasiness Abdominal pain, diarrhea, hepatotoxicity Headache, dizziness Tachycardia	Avoid if pregnant or having surgery within 2 weeks

Abbreviations: CNS, central nervous system; GI, gastrointestinal; HTN, hypertension.
    Data from Refs.[30–51].

CAPSICUM PEPPER (*CAPSICUM FRUTESCENS* OR *ANNUUM*)

Capsicum pepper is ingested or used topically and includes red and cayenne pepper, paprika, and chili.[32] Reported uses include diabetic neuropathy, lower back pain, and postherpetic neuralgia, all of which were rated likely effective. Reported uses that were rated possibly effective include cluster headaches, postoperative and lower back pain, and postoperative nausea.[33]

Adverse reactions include anaphylaxis, abdominal pain, renal and hepatic damage, local burning, edema, erythema, and upper airway reactions. Capsicum pepper should not be used by those with a known hypersensitivity to peppers and those with an upcoming surgery. Caution is advised in patients with a history of bleeding disorders, diabetes mellitus, or hypertension (HTN).[33]

GERMAN CHAMOMILE (*MATRICARIA RECUTITA*)

German chamomile is native to Europe and has been used to treat nervousness, dyspepsia and gastrointestinal (GI) spasms, mild infections, skin conditions, inflammation, and colic (in children). Adverse reactions include anaphylaxis, hypersensitivity and skin reactions, confusion, and drowsiness. German chamomile should not be used in children younger than 2 years; women who are pregnant or breastfeeding; and those with a known hypersensitivity to chrysanthemums, daisies, marigolds, and ragweed. Caution is advised in patients with asthma, hormone-sensitive conditions, and upcoming surgery.[6,34]

CRANBERRY (*VACCINIUM MACROCARPON*)

Cranberry is an evergreen shrub native to North America and has been shown possibly effective in preventing urinary tract infections. Additionally, cranberry has been used to treat benign prostatic hyperplasia (BPH), nephrolithiasis, metabolic syndrome, and influenza. Adverse reactions primarily include abdominal pain, nausea, vomiting, and diarrhea. Cranberry use should be avoided in patients with hypersensitivity to aspirin or other salicylates. Caution should be used in patients with asthma, atrophic gastritis, hypochlorhydria, and nephrolithiasis.[6,35]

ECHINACEA (*ECHINACEA PURPUREA*)

Among the most popular herbs in the United States, the echinacea plant has been used medicinally by Native Americans for hundreds of years. Echinacea is most frequently used as an immune booster and has been shown possibly effective in treating the common cold by reducing symptoms, such as fever, pharyngitis, and cough.[10,16,36] Additional reported uses include anxiety, atopic dermatitis, cough, genital herpes, human papilloma virus, influenza, otitis media, tonsillitis, and warts.[6,36]

Adverse reactions to echinacea include anaphylaxis, angioedema, bronchospasm, hypersensitivity reactions, abdominal discomfort, headache, dizziness, drowsiness, and altered fertility. Echinacea should be avoided in patients with a history of autoimmune disorders. Caution is recommended with patients suffering from atopic conditions and when attempting to conceive a pregnancy.[10,16,36]

EVENING PRIMROSE (*OENOTHERA BIENNIS*)

Evening primrose is a wildflower that has been used to treat attention-deficit/hyperactivity disorder (ADHD), asthma, atopic dermatitis, chronic fatigue syndrome, diabetes mellitus, dry eye syndrome, dyslexia, hepatitis B, hyperlipidemia, liver cancer, multiple sclerosis, obesity, premenstrual syndrome, rheumatoid arthritis, and ulcerative colitis. Adverse reactions include abdominal pain and related symptoms, taste disturbance, acne and skin rash, increased risk of bleeding, dizziness, headache, decreased platelet activity, decreased seizure threshold, and weight gain. Caution should be used in patients with a history of coagulation disorders, schizophrenia, seizure disorder, pregnancy or lactation, or upcoming surgery.[10,37]

FEVERFEW (*TANACETUM PARTHENIUM*)

Feverfew is a member of the daisy family that originated in Europe and is widespread across North America. Ancient Greek physicians were found to have used feverfew to treat menstrual cramps and inflammation. Current reported uses include treatment of allergies, arthritis, psoriasis, fever, headache, tinnitus, vertigo, menstrual irregularities, and migraine headache prophylaxis.[38]

Adverse reactions include abdominal pain and related symptoms, dysgeusia, oral ulcers and gingival bleeding, anxiety, and insomnia. Feverfew should be avoided by pregnant women; patients younger than 18 years; and those with a known hypersensitivity to chrysanthemums, daisies, and marigolds.[38]

FLAX/FLAXSEED OIL (*LINUM USITATISSIMUM*)

Flaxseed, or linseed, is derived from the flax plant and consists of soluble and insoluble fiber; protein; lignans; and α-linoleic acid, an essential omega-3 fatty acid.[16] Flaxseed has long been used for its cardiovascular protective and laxative properties. Current reported uses include hyperlipidemia, HTN, atherosclerosis, diabetes mellitus, obesity, breast cancer, menopausal symptoms, premature labor, and BPH.[39]

Adverse reactions include anaphylactic and hypersensitivity reactions, abdominal pain and related symptoms, hypotension, and mania. Flaxseed should be avoided in patients with history of GI disorders, obstruction, stricture or inflammation, breast uterine or ovarian cancer, uterine fibroids or endometriosis, hypertriglyceridemia, and open wounds. Caution should be used in patients with bipolar disorder, coagulopathies, diabetes mellitus, and hypothyroidism.[6,16,39]

GARLIC (*ALLIUM SATIVUM*)

Used as a food and medicine for thousands of years, garlic is an edible aromatic bulb known for its antiseptic properties. Garlic has also been found to have anticoagulant and antioxidant properties.[16] Evidence supporting the use of garlic is found in multiple systematic reviews and meta-analyses. Current reported uses of garlic include coronary artery disease and prevention, HTN, hyperlipidemia, peripheral vascular disease, upper respiratory tract infections, meningitis, and tinea infections.[16,18,40]

Adverse reactions include anaphylaxis, angioedema, urticaria, abdominal pain and related symptoms, hypotension, and dizziness. Garlic should be avoided in patients with a history of coagulation disorders; recent or upcoming surgery; or hypersensitivity to garlic, lily, hyacinth, tulip, onions, leeks, or chives. Garlic should be used cautiously in patients with diabetes mellitus, GI infections, peptic ulcer disease, or inflammatory bowel disease.[16,40]

GINGER (*ZINGIBER OFFICINALE*)

For thousands of years, ginger has been a popular spice and herbal medicine. Current reported uses include treating nausea, vomiting, dyspepsia, motion sickness, morning sickness, urinary tract dysfunction, osteoarthritis, rheumatoid arthritis, migraines, and to shorten the duration of labor. Research has suggested that the active components of the ginger root include volatile oils and pungent phenol compounds, such as gingerols and shogaols.[10,16,41]

Adverse reactions include abdominal pain and related symptoms, dermatitis, hypoglycemia, central nervous system depression, and arrhythmias. Ginger should be avoided in patients with a history of gallbladder dysfunction, inflammatory bowel disease, or GI obstruction. Caution should be used in patients with a history of cardiac disease, gastric or duodenal ulcers, diabetes mellitus, HTN, hypotension, breastfeeding, or pregnancy.[41]

GINKGO (*GINKGO BILOBA*)

Gingko is one of the best-selling herbal supplements in the United States and is one of the world's oldest tree species. Gingko is generally considered safe when used up to 6 months and is commonly used for mild to moderate depression.[10,13,16,42] Evidence from two randomized trials comparing ginkgo and donepezil found them comparable in patients with mild to moderate Alzheimer disease, supporting the use of ginkgo in the treatment of the disease.[18] Ginkgo has been determined to be possibly effective in the treatment of anxiety, age-related cognitive decline, chemotherapy-related cognitive impairment, dementia, diabetic retinopathy, glaucoma, multiple sclerosis, peripheral arterial disease, premenstrual syndrome, and schizophrenia. Additional reported uses include ADHD, asthma, autism spectrum disorder, chronic obstructive pulmonary disease, depression, cancer prevention, radiation exposure, and the connective tissue disorder Reynaud phenomenon.[42]

Adverse reactions include nausea, vomiting, constipation, diarrhea, xerostomia, arrhythmias, palpitations, transient ischemic attacks, cerebrovascular accidents, edema, increased bleeding risk, hematuria, weakness, restlessness, dizziness, drowsiness, headache, skin hypersensitivity reactions, and Stevens-Johnson syndrome (a disorder of the skin and mucous membranes). Ginkgo should be avoided by patients who are attempting to conceive, are pregnant, or are having surgery within 2 weeks. Caution should be used in patients with a history of bleeding or seizure disorders, diabetes mellitus, or G6PD deficiency.[10,13,42]

GINSENG, AMERICAN (*PANAX QUINQUEFOLIUS*)

American ginseng is one of the most popular herbs in the United States. Research on American ginseng tends to focus on diabetes mellitus, cancer, cold and flu, ADHD, immune system enhancement, and cognition. American ginseng has been rated possibly effective when used in the treatment of diabetes mellitus type 2 and respiratory infections. American ginseng has also been reportedly used for ADHD, breast cancer, cancer-related fatigue, cognitive function, symptoms of menopause, and schizophrenia. The primary associated adverse reaction is headache. American ginseng should be avoided in patients who are pregnant or having surgery within 2 weeks. Caution should be used in patients with bleeding disorders; diabetes mellitus; insomnia; hormone-sensitive conditions; breast, ovarian, or uterine cancers; uterine fibroids; or endometriosis.[6,43]

GINSENG, ASIAN (*PANAX GINSENG*)

Traditional Chinese medicine has incorporated Asian ginseng for thousands of years. Evidence was deemed possibly effective for use related to chronic obstructive pulmonary disease, cognitive function, influenza, multiple sclerosis–related fatigue, sexual arousal, erectile dysfunction, and premature ejaculation. Additionally, Asian ginseng has been used in the treatment of dementia of Alzheimer type, breast cancer, heart failure, cognitive impairment and decline, the common cold, diabetes mellitus type 2, fatigue, fibromyalgia, gallbladder disease, human immunodeficiency virus/AIDS, and HTN.[6,10,44]

Adverse reactions to Asian ginseng include anaphylaxis and skin hypersensitivity reactions, headache, euphoria, insomnia, abdominal pain and related symptoms, cholestatic hepatitis, HTN, hypotension, tachycardia, vaginal bleeding, and amenorrhea. Asian ginseng should be avoided with pediatric patients, pregnant women, organ transplant recipients, and patients with a history of coagulation disorders. Caution should be used in patients with a history of cardiovascular disease, arrhythmias, cerebrovascular disease, autoimmune disorders, endometrial cancer or endometriosis, hormone-sensitive conditions, insomnia, or schizophrenia.[6,44]

GOLDENSEAL (*HYDRASTIS CANADENSIS*)

Goldenseal is frequently combined with echinacea to combat the common cold but there is no evidence to support its efficacy. Similarly, there is no evidence to support its use masking illicit drugs in urine drug screening tests. Adverse reactions include abdominal pain and related complaints, headache, photosensitivity, skin rash, and hyponatremia. Goldenseal should be avoided in infants and women who are pregnant or breastfeeding. Goldenseal should be used with caution in patients with a history of coagulation disorders, diabetes mellitus, HTN, or hypotension.[45]

GREEN TEA (*CAMELLIA SINENSIS*)

Green tea is made from the dried, unoxidized leaves of *Camellia sinensis*. It is reported to contain more antioxidants and beneficial polyphenols than black tea, which represents 78% of worldwide tea consumption. Reported uses of green tea include prevention of cancer, treatment of Parkinson disease, cardiovascular disorders, diabetes mellitus, headaches, fertility disorders, and anxiety.[30]

Adverse reactions include nausea, vomiting, flatulence, abdominal distention, diarrhea, constipation, arrhythmias, palpitations, tachycardia, HTN, dizziness, nervousness, anxiety, restlessness, irritability, insomnia, delirium, rash, urticaria, muscle spasm, and seizures. Green tea should be avoided in patients with hepatic impairment or disease and by women who are pregnant or breastfeeding. Caution should be used with elderly patients, postmenopausal women, patients with a history of cardiovascular disease or arrhythmias, anxiety, diabetes mellitus, HTN, headaches, glaucoma, psychiatric disorders, prostate cancer, renal disease, osteoporosis, and gastric or duodenal ulcers.[16,30]

HAWTHORN (*CRATAEGUS MONOGYNA*)

The leaves, flowers, and berries of the hawthorn plant are used to make this herbal supplement. Reported uses include heart failure, arrhythmias, angina, hyperlipidemia, HTN, atherosclerosis, hypotension, circulatory and functional cardiovascular disorders, anxiety, indigestion, and tapeworm infections. Adverse reactions include nausea, dizziness, agitation, headache, insomnia, palpitations, arrhythmias, circulatory disturbance, and tachycardia. Hawthorn use should be avoided in patients with a known hypersensitivity. Caution should be used with the elderly and with patients concurrently taking central nervous system depressants, cardiovascular drugs, or vasodilatory agents.[46]

KAVA (*PIPER METHYSTICUM*)

Kava, or kava kava, is known for its ceremonial use and relaxing qualities. Reported uses include anxiety and depressive disorders, stress, insomnia, psychosis, Parkinson disease, epilepsy, migraine headaches, and musculoskeletal pain. Adverse effects include hepatotoxicity, hepatic failure, hepatitis, cirrhosis, weight loss, skin hypersensitivity reactions, mydriasis, ocular motor equilibrium and visual accommodation disturbances, headache, motor reflex impairment, and dyskinesia. Kava should be avoided in patients who are pregnant or breastfeeding, have a history of or acute hepatitis, long-term ethanol use, chronic lung disease, Parkinson disease, or who are taking concurrent central nervous system depressants or hepatotoxic drugs. Caution should be used in patients suffering from depressive disorders.[6,10,47]

MILK THISTLE (*SILYBUM MARIANUM*)

Milk thistle is native to the Mediterranean and has long been used as an herbal remedy for liver (alcoholic and viral hepatitis), kidney, and gallbladder problems; cancer; and mushroom poisoning. Milk thistle is reported to be possibly effective in the treatment of diabetes mellitus and dyspepsia. Milk thistle is also used in the treatment of liver disease, hepatitis B and C, acne, dementia of Alzheimer type, diabetes mellitus, diabetic nephropathy, multiple sclerosis, Parkinson disease, prostate cancer, and ulcerative colitis.[48]

Adverse reactions include anaphylaxis or hypersensitivity reactions, abdominal pain and related symptoms, loss of appetite, weakness, rash, pruritus, eczema, and dysgeusia. Milk thistle should be avoided in patients with breast, ovarian, or uterine cancers; endometriosis; uterine fibroids; hormone-sensitive conditions; or a known hypersensitivity to chrysanthemums, daisies, or marigolds. Caution should be used in patients with diabetes mellitus.[10,16,48]

SAW PALMETTO (*SERENOA REPENS*)

Saw palmetto is a fan palm with berries that has been used by men since the early 1900s to treat urinary tract problems, increase sperm production, and boost libido. More recently, saw palmetto has been found to be possibly effective when used before transurethral resection of the prostate. Other reported uses include BPH, hypotonic bladder, and chronic prostatitis.[13,16,49]

Adverse effects include abdominal pain and related symptoms, hepatitis, arrhythmias, angina, congestive heart failure, HTN, hypotension, myocardial infarction, tachycardia, dyspnea, headache, dizziness, weakness, myalgias, insomnia, and rhabdomyolysis. Additional adverse effects include testicular pain, urinary tract infection, decreased libido, and erectile dysfunction. Saw palmetto should be avoided by women who are pregnant or breastfeeding and is no longer recommended to manage symptoms of BPH. Caution should be used in patients with coagulation disorders or hormone-sensitive conditions.[16,19,49]

ST. JOHN'S WORT (*HYPERICUM PERFORATUM*)

St. John's wort is a flowering plant that is considered a noxious weed in seven US states and two Canadian provinces; however, it is one of the most frequently used herbal supplements. Extracts are available in multiple forms, including capsules, tinctures, and topical preparations. Primarily, St. John's wort has been studied in relation to major depressive disorder and has been deemed likely effective. It has been found to be possibly effective in the treatment of menopausal symptoms, somatoform disorders, and wound healing. Additional reported uses include ADHD, angioplasty, anxiety, glioma, Crigler-Najjar syndrome, migraine headaches, obsessive-compulsive disorder, polycystic ovary syndrome, premenstrual syndrome, plaque psoriasis, seasonal affective disorder, and smoking cessation.[10,13,16,50]

St. John's wort may have an effect on serotonin levels and precipitate serotonin syndrome in patients taking selective serotonin reuptake inhibitors (SSRIs). Patients taking St. John's wort should be tapered off when initiating an SSRI and educated against concurrent use of St. John's wort and SSRIs.[24] St. John's wort has also been shown to interact with tricyclic antidepressants and benzodiazepines.[6,24,50]

Additional adverse effects include anorexia, nausea, vomiting, diarrhea, constipation, dyspepsia, hypoglycemia, xerostomia, agitation, dizziness, anxiety, fatigue, hypomania, irritability, lethargy, panic attacks, psychosis, restlessness, suicidal or homicidal ideation, vivid dreams, tremor, and withdrawal-like symptoms. Muscle pain, joint stiffness, pruritus, jaundice, palpitations, HTN, tachycardia, and sexual dysfunction have also been reported. St. John's wort should be avoided if having surgery within 2 weeks and by women having difficulty conceiving a pregnancy. Caution should be used with patients suffering from dementia of Alzheimer type, bipolar disorder, depression, schizophrenia, or with concurrent use of anesthesia or a dose greater than 2 g per day.[6,16,19,50]

VALERIAN (*VALERIANA OFFICINALIS*)

Valerian is a perennial plant native to Europe whose root is used to create herbal supplements. Reported uses that were judged possibly effective include insomnia and menopausal symptoms. Valerian is also used in the treatment of anxiety, depression, dysmenorrhea, premenstrual syndrome, and stress.[51] Adverse reactions include abdominal pain and related GI symptoms, agitation, excitability, drowsiness, sedation, headache, dizziness, and tachycardia. Valerian should be avoided within 2 weeks of surgery and by women who are pregnant or breastfeeding.[51]

RESOURCES

To promote safe use and minimize adverse reactions and herb-drug interactions, health care providers should educate themselves and patients on potential interactions between prescribed medications and herbal supplements. In addition there are free and subscription drug databases that index herbal supplements and provide interaction checkers, such as Epocrates or Natural Medicines. Epocrates is a comprehensive database for finding information about medications, including uses, dosing, contraindications, reactions, interactions, pregnancy, pharmacology, and more. In addition, Epocrates includes herbal supplements and diseases in its database. Natural Medicines provides a database of dietary supplements that claims to be impartial and not supported by interest groups, professional organizations, or product manufacturers. Additional resources include nonprofit organizations, such as the American Botanic Council, and independent companies, including the American Herbalist Guild. To encourage reporting of adverse effects of herb-drug interactions, the FDA maintains an online reporting mechanism for health care providers, consumers, and industry members via the Safety Reporting Portal at the Department of Health and Human Services Web site.[2,52]

The FDA Office of Dietary Supplements is a branch of the National Institutes of Health concerned with promoting scientific research related to dietary supplements. The Office of Dietary Supplements maintains dietary supplement fact sheets and a dietary supplement label database. Formerly known as the National Center for Complementary and Alternative Medicine, the National Center for Complementary and Integrative Health is a branch of the National Institutes of Health responsible for scientific research on the diverse medical and health care systems, practices, and products that are not generally considered part of conventional medicine. The National Center for Complementary and Integrative Health provides a variety of educational materials for consumers and health care providers, including herbs at a glance, literature and Cochrane reviews, and AHRQ evidence reports. Refer to **Table 3** for details and links to available resources.[20,53,54]

Table 3
Resources for providers and consumers

Resource/Link	About	Comments
Allied and Complementary Database (AMED)[a] health.ebsco.com/products/amed-the-allied-and-complementary-medicine-database	Produced by the Health Care Information Service of the British Library	Specialized bibliographic database about alternative and allied therapies and related subjects
American Botanic Council herbalgram.org	Independent, nonprofit research and education organization	News, herbal library, programs, services, and support
Epocrates[a] epocrates.com	Mobile medical reference app owned by Athena Health	Drug and dietary supplement monographs, interaction check
NIH National Center for Complementary and Integrative Health[b] nccih.nih.gov	Branch of NIH responsible for scientific research on health care systems, practices, and products not generally considered part of conventional medicine	Herbs at a glance, literature and Cochrane reviews, AHRQ evidence reports, interactive education modules
NIH Office of Dietary Supplements ods.od.nih.gov	Branch of NIH concerned with promoting scientific research related to dietary supplements	Dietary supplement fact sheets and label database
Natural Medicines[a] http://trchealthcare.com/natural-medicines/	TRC Healthcare is a provider of evidence-based drug therapy recommendations to pharmacists, physicians, medical personnel, and consumers	Database of dietary supplements, interaction check
US Food and Drug Administration https://www.fda.gov/food/dietary-supplements/how-report-problem-dietary-supplements safetyreporting.hhs.gov	Federal government regulatory agency	Report a problem with dietary supplements
US Pharmacopeia http://usp.org/	Nonprofit organization aiming to improve global health through public standards and programs that help ensure the quality, safety, and benefit of medicines and foods	Herbal medicines compendium, reference standards, education programs

Abbreviation: NIH, National Institutes of Health.
[a] Subscription or fee may be required to access all content.
[b] Formerly known as the National Center for Complementary and Alternative Medicine.

SUMMARY

Herbal supplements are commonly used yet poorly understood.[13,20] To combat the lack of available scientific evidence and variable research findings, efforts to promote scientific research are needed. Evidence demonstrating the efficacy and safety of herbal supplements will help to minimize adverse effects, prevent herbal-drug interactions, and improve patient outcomes. In addition, evidence will inform the development of education strategies for health care providers and consumers. Finally, increased attention to regulatory standards and quality assurance for herbal supplements will serve to ensure their safe and effective use.[4,16,19]

CLINICS CARE POINTS

- As the use of herbal supplements and medications continues to increase, healthcare providers must educate themselves on potential adverse reactions and interactions with prescribed medications.
- Because herbal supplements and medication are not regulated by the FDA, limited evidence exists to guide their use in clinical practice.
- Classes of drugs associated with herbal supplement and medication interactions include anticoagulants, cardiovascular agents, diabetes drugs, and HIV drugs.
- Healthcare providers should routinely ask patients about herbal supplement and medication use.

REFERENCES

1. US Food & Drug Administration. Botanical drug development: guidance for industry. U.S. Department of Health and Human Services; 2016. Available at: https://www.fda.gov/%20downloads/Drugs/Guidances/UCM458484.pdf. Accessed June 20, 2020.
2. National Institutes of Health. Dietary and Herbal Supplements. Office of Dietary Supplements. Available at: https://www.nccih.nih.gov/health/dietary-and-herbal-supplements. Accessed June 29, 2020.
3. National Institutes of Health. Botanical Dietary Supplements. Office of Dietary Supplements. Available at: https://ods.od.nih.gov/factsheets/BotanicalBackground-HealthProfessional. Accessed June 29, 2020.
4. Govindaraghavan S, Sucher NJ. Quality assessment of medicinal herbs and their extracts: criteria and prerequisites for consistent safety and efficacy of herbal medicines. Epilepsy Behav 2015;52:363–71.
5. Smith T, Gillespie M, Eckl V, et al. Herbal supplement sales in US increase by 9.4% in 2018. Herbalgram 2019;123:62–73. Available at: http://cms.herbalgram.org/herbalgram/issue123/files/HG123-HMR.pdf.
6. Johns Hopkins Medicine. Herbal Medicine. Available at: https://www.hopkinsmedicine.org/health/wellness-and-prevention/herbal-medicine. Accessed June 1, 2020.
7. Lenssen KG, Bast A, de Boer A. International perspectives on substantiating the efficacy of herbal dietary supplements and herbal medicines through evidence on traditional use. Compr Rev Food Sci Food Saf 2019;18:910–22.
8. US Food and Drug Administration. Development & Approval Process - Drugs. Available at: https://www.fda.gov/drugs/development-approval-process-drugs. Accessed June 30, 2020.
9. Public Law 103-417 Dietary Supplement Health and Education Act of 1994. Text from: United States Public Laws. LexisNexis Congressional. Available at: https://www.fda.

gov/food/dietary-supplements/how-report-problem-dietary-supplements. Accessed June 30, 2020.

10. Dasgupta A. Anti-inflammatory herbal supplements. In: Actor JK, Smith KC, editors. Translational inflammation. Alpharetta (GA): Elsevier; 2019. p. 69–91.

11. Cohen PA, Benner C, McCormick D. Use of a pharmaceutically adulterated dietary supplement, Pai You Guo, among Brazilian-born women in the United States. J Gen Intern Med 2012;27(1):51–6.

12. Cohen PA, Maller G, DeSouza R, et al. Presence of banned drugs in dietary supplements following FDA recalls. JAMA 2014;312(16):1691–3. Available at: https://jamanetwork.com/journals/jama/article-abstract/1917421.

13. Pereira K. Herbal supplements: widely used, poorly understood. Plast Surg Nurs 2016;46(2):54–9.

14. US Food and Drug Administration. Background: final rule for current good manufacturing practices for dietary supplements. Available at: https://wayback.archive-it.org/7993/20170406030847/https://www.fda.gov/Food/GuidanceRegulation/CGMP/ucm110863.htm. Accessed June 30, 2020.

15. Asher GN, Corbett AH, Hawke RL. Common herbal dietary supplement-drug interactions. Am Fam Physician 2017;96(2):101–7. Available at: https://www.aafp.org/afp/2017/0715/p101.html.

16. Pruitt R, Lemanski A, Carroll A. Herbal supplements: research findings and safety. Nurse Pract 2018;43(5):32–43.

17. Parveen A, Parveen B, Parveen R, et al. Challenges and guidelines for clinical trials of herbal drugs. J Pharm Bioallied Sci 2015;7(4):329. Available at: https://www.ncbi.nlm.nih.gov/pmc/articles/PMC4678978/.

18. Schaffer SD, Yoon S, Curry K. Herbal supplements for health promotion and disease prevention. Nurse Pract 2016;41(10):39–48.

19. Rashrash M, Schommer JC, Brown LM. Prevalence and predictors of herbal medicine use among adults in the United States. J Patient Exp 2017 Sep;4(3):108–13.

20. Brown AC. An overview of herb and dietary supplement efficacy, safety and government regulations in the United States with suggested improvements. Part 1 of 5 series. Food Chem Toxicol 2017;107:449–71.

21. Swann JP. The history of efforts to regulate dietary supplements in the USA. Drug Test Anal 2016;8:271–82.

22. Long J. FDA GMP inspectors cite 70% of dietary supplement firms. Natural Products Insider Website. Available at: https://www.naturalproductsinsider.com/fda-gmp-inspectors-cite-70-dietary-supplement-firms. Accessed June 30, 2020.

23. Jou J, Johnson PJ. Non-disclosure of complementary and alternative medicine use to primary care physicians: findings from the 2012 national health interview survey. JAMA 2016;176(4):545–55. Available at: https://jamanetwork.com/journals/jamainternalmedicine/article-abstract/2500061.

24. Gardiner P, Phillips R, Shaughnessy AF. Herbal and dietary supplement-drug interactions in patients with chronic illnesses. Am Fam Physician 2008;77(1):73–8. Available at: https://www.aafp.org/afp/2008/0101/p73.html.

25. Kaye AD. Critical care medicine and the emerging challenges of dietary supplements, including herbal products. Crit Care Med 2014;42(4):1014–6.

26. Saper RB. Overview of herbal medicine and dietary supplements. In: UpToDate. 2020. Available at: http://www.uptodate.com. Accessed June 30, 2020.

27. de Souza Silva JE, Souza CA, da Silva TB, et al. Use of herbal medicines by elderly patients: a systematic review. Arch Gerontol Geriatr Suppl 2014;59(2):227–33.

28. Amer MR, Cipriano GC, Venci JV, et al. Safety of popular herbal supplements in lactating women. J Hum Lact 2015;31(3):348–53.

29. Palleria C, Di Paolo A, Giofre C, et al. Pharmacokinetic drug-drug interaction and their implication in clinical management. J Res Med Sci 2013;18(7):601–10. Available at: https://www.ncbi.nlm.nih.gov/pmc/articles/PMC3897029/.

30. Green tea (Camellia sinensis). Epocrates Version. 20.6 [iPad]. Epocrates, Inc, San Francisco (CA). Available at: https://online.epocrates.com/. Accessed June 15, 2020.

31. TRC Healthcare. Alternative medication effectiveness rating definitions. Epocrates Version. 20.6 [iPad]. Epocrates, Inc, San Francisco (CA). Available at: https://online.epocrates.com/. Accessed June 15, 2020.

32. Farkas J, Mohacsi-Farkas C. Foods, materials, technologies and risks. Encyclopedia of Food Safety. Alpharetta (GA): Elsevier; 2014.

33. Capsicum frutescens [monograph]. Epocrates Version. 20.6 [iPad]. Epocrates, Inc, San Francisco (CA). Available at: https://online.epocrates.com/. Accessed June 15, 2020.

34. Chamomile, German[monograph]. Epocrates Version. 20.6 [iPad]. Epocrates, Inc, San Francisco (CA). Available at: https://online.epocrates.com/. Accessed June 15, 2020.

35. Cranberry [monograph]. Epocrates Version. 20.6 [iPad]. Epocrates, Inc, San Francisco (CA). Available at: https://online.epocrates.com/. Accessed June 15, 2020.

36. Echinacea purpurea [monograph]. Epocrates Version. 20.6 [iPad]. Epocrates, Inc, San Francisco (CA). Available at: https://online.epocrates.com/. Accessed June 15, 2020.

37. Evening Primrose Oil (Oenothera biennis) [monograph]. Epocrates Version. 20.6 [iPad]. Epocrates, Inc, San Francisco (CA). Available at: https://online.epocrates.com/. Accessed June 15, 2020.

38. Feverfew (Tanacetum parthenium). Epocrates Version. 20.6 [iPad]. Epocrates, Inc, San Francisco (CA). Available at: https://online.epocrates.com/. Accessed June 15, 2020.

39. Flaxseed (Linum usitatissimum) Epocrates Version. 20.6 [iPad]. Epocrates, Inc, San Francisco (CA). Available at: https://online.epocrates.com/. Accessed June 15, 2020.

40. Garlic (Allium sativum). Epocrates Version. 20.6 [iPad]. Epocrates, Inc, San Francisco (CA). Available at: https://online.epocrates.com/. Accessed June 15, 2020.

41. Ginger (Zingiber officinale). Epocrates Version. 20.6 [iPad]. Epocrates, Inc, San Francisco, CA. Available at: https://online.epocrates.com/. Accessed June 15, 2020.

42. Gingko (Gingko biloba). Epocrates Version. 20.6 [iPad]. Epocrates, Inc, San Francisco, CA. Available at: https://online.epocrates.com/. Accessed June 15, 2020.

43. Ginseng, American (Panax quinquefolius). Epocrates Version. 20.6 [iPad]. Epocrates, Inc, San Francisco, CA. Available at: https://online.epocrates.com/. Accessed June 15, 2020.

44. Ginseng, Asian (Panax ginseng). Epocrates Version. 20.6 [iPad]. Epocrates, Inc, San Francisco, CA. Available at: https://online.epocrates.com/. Accessed June 15, 2020.

45. Goldenseal (Hydrastis canadensis). Epocrates Version. 20.6 [iPad]. Epocrates, Inc, San Francisco, CA. Available at: https://online.epocrates.com/. Accessed June 15, 2020.

46. Hawthorn (Crataegus spp.). Epocrates Version. 20.6 [iPad]. Epocrates, Inc, San Francisco, CA. Available at: https://online.epocrates.com/. Accessed June 15, 2020.

47. Kava (Piper methysticum). Epocrates Version. 20.6 [iPad]. Epocrates, Inc, San Francisco, CA. Available at: https://online.epocrates.com/. Accessed June 15, 2020.

48. Milk thistle (Silybum marianum). Epocrates Version. 20.6 [iPad]. Epocrates, Inc, San Francisco, CA. Available at: https://online.epocrates.com/. Accessed June 15, 2020.

49. Saw palmetto (Serenoa repens). Epocrates Version. 20.6 [iPad]. Epocrates, Inc, San Francisco, CA. Available at: https://online.epocrates.com/. Accessed June 15, 2020.

50. St. John's wort (Hypericum perforatum). Epocrates Version. 20.6 [iPad]. Epocrates, Inc, San Francisco, CA. Available at: https://online.epocrates.com/. Accessed June 15, 2020.

51. Valerian (Valeriana officinalis). Epocrates Version. 20.6 [iPad]. Epocrates, Inc, San Francisco, CA. Available at: https://online.epocrates.com/. Accessed June 15, 2020.

52. US Food and Drug Administration. How to report a problem with dietary supplements. Available at: https://www.fda.gov/food/dietary-supplements/how-report-problem-dietary-supplements. Accessed June 15, 2020.

53. National Institutes of Health. What does NCCIH do? NCCIH. Available at: https://www.nccih.nih.gov/. Accessed June 15, 2020.

54. National Institutes of Health. Using Dietary Supplements Wisely. Office of Dietary Supplements. Available at: https://www.nccih.nih.gov/health/using-dietary-supplements-wisely. Accessed June 29, 2020.

The Role of Vitamin B6 in Women's Health

Amy S.D. Lee, DNP, ARNP, WHNP-BC

KEYWORDS

- Vitamins • Women's health • Complementary medicine • Vitamin B6 • Pyroxidine

KEY POINTS

- Vitamin B6, or pyroxidine, is a water-soluble vitamin that serves as a cofactor for 140 to 150 cellular reactions.
- Women are particularly susceptible to various health issues.
- The cellular reactions facilitated by vitamin B6 have implications for the health issues faced by women.
- Consideration of vitamin B6 in women's health suggests a benefit for supplementation of vitamin B6.

INTRODUCTION

Vitamin B6, also known as pyroxidine, is a central molecule in the cells of living organisms.[1] As a cofactor in over 140 to 150 biochemical reactions in the cell, it regulates basic cellular metabolism and affects overall physiology.[1,2] It is an essential coenzyme for various catabolic and anabolic processes[3] including amino acid, glucose, and lipid metabolism.[4]

The vitamin contains 6 chemically related compounds that all contain pyridine as their core.[1] They are modified at their fourth position to create 3 groups: pyridoxamine, pyridoxine, and pyridoxal.[1] The water-soluble vitamin is not synthesized in the body but must be ingested from various foods that include certain animal products, beans, nuts, potatoes, fruits, and vegetables. The 3 groups making up the vitamin are dephosphorylated in the intestine and then rephosphorylated by the liver into the biologically active form of B6 called pyridoxal 5' -phosphate (PLP).[1,2] The liver exports PLP through a tightly regulated system that maintains a relatively constant rate in the blood bound to albumin, where it is transported to cells and tissues and crosses the blood/brain barrier. It is there that it serves as a cofactor for the more than 150 enzymes catalyzing a range of activities.[1]

Most of the vitamin B6 reactions are related to amino acid biosynthesis and catabolism. However, it also contributes to fatty acid biosynthesis,[1] gluconeogenesis, and

Capstone College of Nursing, University of Alabama, 650 University Boulevard East, Tuscaloosa, AL 35401, USA
E-mail address: adlee5@ua.edu

Nurs Clin N Am 56 (2021) 23–32
https://doi.org/10.1016/j.cnur.2020.10.002
0029-6465/21/© 2020 Elsevier Inc. All rights reserved.

heme and neurotransmitter biosynthesis.[2] In addition to these roles as a cofactor, the vitamin has been considered to be a scavenger of reactive oxygen species, a metal chelator, and a chaperone in the enzyme folding process.[1,2] It is through these processes that the suggestion of relief for various conditions begins to surface.

Vitamin B6 deficiency in the modern diet is thought to be rare.[2] However, it can be seen with certain medications, excessive alcohol consumption, severe renal disease, some malabsorption syndromes, and certain genetic disorders, as well as in adults older than 45 years old.[1] The recommended daily allowance is met with consumption of 1.3 to 1.7 mg daily or 2 mg daily in lactating women. Deficiency is uncommon in the average balanced diet of the healthy person in developed countries. If documented vitamin B6 deficiency does occur as reflected by low serum PLP levels, it has been associated with dermatitis, microcytic anemia, electroencephalographic abnormalities, decreased immune function, convulsive seizures, depression, and confusion.[1] Although correcting deficits is certainly beneficial, increasing serum PLP levels above sufficient has not demonstrated any additional benefit.[5] However, vitamin B6 supplementation overdosage is difficult to achieve, with neurologic side effects seen only in profoundly high supplemental doses for prolonged periods of time (2000–6000 mg/d for 2–40 months). With the recommended tolerable supplemental daily dose of 100 mg daily, it is unlikely there would be any ill effects while the potential for benefit exists if a deficit is corrected through supplementation.[1]

Women are affected by certain health issues that are part of the array of disorders potentially alleviated through vitamin B6 supplementation. Some health issues affecting women are unique to women alone, while others have particular unique implications for women.[6] It is this understanding that brings the necessity to look closer at the role of vitamin B6 and the health of women.

DISCUSSION
Cognitive Effects

Depression/anxiety/stress
Depression is a common but serious mood disorder that causes severe symptoms affecting daily living activities like sleeping, eating, or working.[7] Depression is more common in women than men. This is likely because of certain factors that are unique to women that are biological, hormonal, or social. Recent evidence on depression suggests that this is a combination of genetic, biological, environmental, and psychological factors. Although sadness may be a part of depression, other symptoms include physical manifestations, trouble sleeping, trouble waking, fatigue, and difficulty in thoughts. Most people need treatment to overcome depression.[7] Depression has significant implications for health care costs, personal costs, and societal costs, with around 350 million people affected worldwide. Although only about 39% of those with depression will seek treatment, up to 50% of those who achieve remission will suffer recurrent depression. The need for alternative and supplemental mechanisms to aid in the treatment and prevention of recurrent depression is valuable.[8]

Low vitamin B6 levels are known to be associated with depressive symptoms.[8] Nutrient deficiencies as a role in depression are recognized as a contributor. Malnutrition may result from inadequate dietary intake caused by age-related conditions, metabolic dysregulation, poor nutrient absorption, polypharmacy, or social stressors. Severe stress and stressful life events have been found to be associated with depression and recurrence of depression. Stress influences the adrenal glands to increase cortisol production. That increased cortisol affects insulin and glucose balance that further affects the appetite resulting in nutritional deficits.[8] Vitamin B6 exerts modulatory effects on the neurotransmitters that affect depression and anxiety while reducing the peripheral effect of corticosteroid release that moderates the stress response.[9] Arévalo and colleagues[8] found that vitamin B6 supplementation in depressed older patients resulted in lower depressive symptoms consistent with previous studies. This result was persistent over time and through control for confounding variables. Vitamin B6 supplementation for the relief of depression, anxiety, and stress has been shown to be beneficial.[8,9]

Premenstrual syndrome

Premenstrual Syndrome (PMS) refers to a constellation of psychological and physical symptoms that occur during the late luteal phase of the menstrual cycle.[10] PMS is common,[7] with some estimates predicting it affects approximately 20% to 30% of all women,[11] while other sources indicate up to 85% of women may have experienced at least 1 PMS symptom at some point.[10] PMS symptoms are usually mild,[7] but around 2.5% to 3% of women will have a severe form of PMS referred to as premenstrual dysphoric disorder (PMDD).[10] Psychological symptoms of PMS may include anxiety, depression, mood instability, fatigue, and impaired thinking, while physical symptoms may include breast and abdominal swelling and tenderness, acne, headache, backache, sleep disturbances, and increased appetite.[10]

Studies have shown vitamin B6 supplementation to demonstrate a beneficial effect on PMS symptoms. Kashanian[12] demonstrated an improvement in physical symptoms like edema, bloating, and heart palpitations, as well as psychological symptoms like irritability, anxiety, food cravings, and disruptions in thought, while Chou[13] showed a reduction in psychological symptoms such as anxiety, fatigue, sleep disturbances, and difficulty in thinking. Panay[14] showed an improvement in overall PMS symptoms with supplementation of vitamin B6 in a systematic review of 9 published studies. Finally, Masoumi and colleagues[10] demonstrated that using a combination of vitamin B6 and calcium resulted in an overall reduction in PMS symptoms including both psychological and physical symptoms. Based on these findings, they recommend supplementation for symptom relief in the PMS patient.[10]

Perinatal depression

Perinatal depression is a serious mood disorder that can affect women during pregnancy or during the postpartum period.[7] It may include feelings of sadness, anxiety, and fatigue that can interfere with the ability to perform daily tasks including self, infant, and family care.[7] It is estimated that between 13% and 20% of pregnant women will experience perinatal depression. Symptoms of perinatal depression may include mood disturbances, sleep and appetite disorders, psychosomatic complaints, fatigue, difficulty concentrating, and general lack of joy.[15]

Shibata and colleagues[16] found that serum PLP levels declined significantly in the second and third trimesters of pregnancy and did not return to first trimester levels until 1 month after delivery. Vitamin B6 supplementation in pregnancy has been shown to be safe with no adverse effects on pregnancy outcomes, even when given at elevated doses.[15] Khodaded and colleagues[15] supplemented women at risk for perinatal depression with 40 mg of vitamin B6 twice daily and demonstrated a significant reduction score in depression scores. They concluded that vitamin B6 supplementation in the third trimester of pregnancy may reduce perinatal depression without further adverse risk to the pregnancy or fetus.[15]

Cognitive decline

Alzheimer disease is a fatal disease of progressive dementia and cognitive decline.[17] Around two-thirds of US patients with Alzheimer disease are women, with the lifetime risk of Alzheimer disease for women being 1 in 5. Women in their 60s are twice as likely to develop Alzheimer disease as breast cancer.[17] Vitamin B6 is a coenzyme for many of the processes that have been indicated in brain health and aging.[4] As an integral contributor to the synthesis of several important neurotransmitters, vitamin B6 is thought to play a key role in the support of cognitive function. Inversely, vitamin B6 deficiency has been targeted as a modifiable risk factor in the prevention of cognitive decline and Alzheimer disease.[4]

Palacios and colleagues[4] followed older adults over a 2-year period and found that lower PLP levels correlated with cognitive decline. This was similar to findings by Tucker and colleagues[18] and Hughes and colleagues,[19] who both found correlations between plasma vitamin B6 levels and cognitive decline. Palacios and colleagues[4] incidentally also found that in their older population studied, 12% of patients were deficient, and 17% had insufficient levels of vitamin B6. While they did not study the effect of vitamin B6 supplementation on cognitive decline, the deficient and insufficient amounts found in their population infer value for supplementation in this population.[4]

Metabolic and Inflammatory Processes

Cancer: breast, colorectal

Because of the role of vitamin B6 as a coenzyme in amino acid metabolism, there has been a growing body of evidence into the vitamin's anti-inflammatory and antioxidant properties.[20] It is through these properties that the preventive possibilities in relation to certain malignancies become a consideration.[20] Certain malignancies where inflammation is believed to play a role in the pathogenesis or progression have been specifically targeted and investigated including colon and breast cancer.[2] Of US women, 1 in 8 will develop breast cancer over their lifetime, with breast cancer being the most common cancer affecting women except for skin cancer. Only 1 in 1000 men will develop breast cancer.[21] Around 1 in 24 women will develop colon cancer over their lifetime. Although colon cancer risk is slightly higher in men, it is the third most commonly diagnosed cancer in men and women combined and the second most common cancer-related cause for death in men and women combined.[22] Vitamin B6 supplementation has been shown to improve some immunologic and inflammatory parameters in those with deficiencies.[2]

Agnoli and colleagues[3] found that breast cancer risk of menopausal women and premenopausal women decreased with elevated plasma vitamin B6 levels. They also found that increased levels of plasma vitamin B6 among women who drank more than 7 g/d of alcohol significantly lowered their breast cancer risk. They concluded that higher plasma vitamin B6 levels may decrease breast cancer risk in all women, and particularly in women who are heavy alcohol drinkers.[3] This was similarly consistent with Lurie and colleagues,[23] who found that women with high vitamin B6 levels had lowered breast cancer risk.

Jia, Wang, and Tian[24] completed a meta-analysis of 10 studies looking at vitamin B6 and colorectal cancer risk. They found a nonsignificant but present association between vitamin B6 intake and a decrease in colorectal cancer risk. But they also found that increasing doses of vitamin B6 supplementation resulted in a significant decrease in colorectal cancer risk.[24] Gylling and colleagues[5] found that vitamin B6 deficiency was associated with a clear increase in the risk of colorectal cancer, with indicators that the inflammatory and oxidative properties play a role in tumor progression. They did not find any indication that vitamin B6 levels above sufficient were beneficial.[5]

Chronic disease: cardiovascular disease, insulin, and glucose dysfunction

The inflammatory and immune pathways that provide the evidence for cancer prevention also lead to the same considerations for other chronic diseases mediated by the same factors.[20] Low plasma vitamin B6 levels have been associated with cardiovascular disease (CVD)[2,25] and insulin resistance.[25] CVD is the leading cause of death for women in the United States, with 1 of 16 US women over the age of 20 affected by CVD.[26] Diabetes is a risk factor for CVD.[26] Insulin resistance develops when cells do not respond properly to insulin, prompting the pancreas to produce more insulin in order to maintain normal glucose levels. Over time, the pancreas fails to produce enough insulin, and glucose levels increase until diabetes is present. Truncal or abdominal obesity appears to be a causative factor for insulin resistance. Inflammation created by the fat cells in the abdomen contribute to insulin resistance, diabetes, and CVD.[27] Diabetes increases the risk of CVD in women fourfold, whereas this in only true twofold in men. Furthermore, heart attack outcomes and diabetes-related outcomes for women are worse than those for men.[28]

Liu and colleagues[25] found that in mice fed a high-fat diet, vitamin B6 decreased endothelial dysfunction, enhanced insulin sensitivity, and prevented hepatic lipid accumulation. They also included an investigation of human subjects with known nonalcoholic fatty liver disease (NAFLD) compared with healthy subjects. They found that those with NAFLD demonstrated lower levels of vitamin B6. Endothelial dysfunction is a hallmark of CVD, while insulin resistance holds the risk for diabetes and CVD. NAFLD is a component of the metabolic syndrome associated with CVD, insulin resistance, and diabetes. They confirmed the protective effect of vitamin B6 on glucose metabolism and the vascular endothelium, as well as the prevention of hepatic lipid accumulation. They were able to report that vitamin B6 administration prevented endothelial dysfunction, insulin resistance, and hepatic lipid accumulation.[25]

Pregnancy

Pregnancy outcomes

Adequate maternal vitamin B6 levels are thought to be critical to healthy pregnancy outcomes.[29] Because adequate levels need to be present from conception throughout pregnancy, it is important for women to maintain sufficient vitamin B6 levels during the reproductive years.[29] Complications of pregnancy are those health problems that occur during pregnancy, resulting in poor pregnancy outcomes. This may affect the mother, the fetus, or both. Pregnancy loss prior to 20 weeks of pregnancy occurs in around 20% of pregnancies often before a woman even knows she is pregnant. Maternal issues after 20 weeks include preeclampsia, a condition that results in high blood pressure and problems for the kidneys and other organs. Fetal problems include a baby that may be smaller than normal for gestational age.[30]

A meta-analysis performed by Ho and colleagues[29] found evidence that supplementation with vitamin B6 in pregnancy resulted in higher infant birth weights[31] and lower rates of preeclampsia,[32] while those with lower PLP levels exhibited lower infant Apgar scores[33,34] and higher incidence of early pregnancy loss.[35] Ho and colleagues[29] sought to determine the prevalence of suboptimal vitamin B6 levels and vitamin B6 deficiency in their local population of healthy young adult women to determine if supplementation should be a general recommendation for reproductive-aged women. They determined that 12.4% of women in their study population had either suboptimal vitamin B6 levels or were vitamin B6 deficient. They found that the use of supplemental vitamin B6 was a strong predictor of PLP concentration and noted that vitamin B6 is crucial for healthy pregnancy outcomes.[29]

Nausea/vomiting

Nausea and vomiting in pregnancy are among the most common early pregnancy complaints.[36] Up to 85% of pregnant women will experience nausea and vomiting, while around 3% will have the most severe form known as hyperemesis gravidarum.[37] Hyperemesis gravidarum is characterized by weight loss, reduced appetite, dehydration, and nausea with vomiting that do not resolve.[30] Women with hyperemesis gravidarum can have both significant adverse physical and psychological sequelae.[37] Early treatment of nausea and vomiting in pregnancy is recommended to prevent progression into hyperemesis gravidarum.[38] According to the American College of Obstetricians and Gynecologists (ACOG),[38] vitamin B6 with or without the addition of the drug doxylamine is considered first-line pharmacotherapeutic treatment of nausea and vomiting in pregnancy.

A systematic review conducted by McParlin and colleagues.[37] found that in 35 randomized control trials (RCTs), vitamin B6 alone (for mild symptoms) and vitamin B6 combined with the drug doxylamine (for moderate symptoms) demonstrated improvement in symptoms compared with placebo. One RCT demonstrated an improvement in moderate-to-severe symptoms when taken prophylactically.[37] Festin[39] also conducted a systematic review to determine the effectiveness of treatments for nausea and vomiting in pregnancy and hyperemesis gravidarum. They found that vitamin B6 was likely to be effective in treating nausea and vomiting in early pregnancy, with evidence particularly supportive of nausea relief. ACOG[38] notes that vitamin B6 alone or in combination with doxylamine has been shown to be safe in pregnancy in numerous studies. Based on the demonstrated effectiveness of Vitamin B6 alone or in combination with doxylamine in the reduction of nausea and vomiting in pregnancy and the safe tolerability of vitamin B6 among pregnant women, ACOG[38] recommends vitamin B6 alone or in combination with doxylamine as first-line treatment for nausea and vomiting in pregnancy.

Menopause

Hot flashes

The menopausal transition is that point in a woman's life when the hormone production from the ovaries declines.[40] This decline in hormonal production results in changes in the menstrual cycle that ultimately culminate in cessation of menses altogether and the phase of life known as menopause. The menopausal transition varies but usually lasts for anywhere from 7 to 14 years. During this time, the woman may experience a variety of symptoms that may be mild or severe. Hot flashes are a common symptom of the menopausal transition.[40] Hot flashes are described as a sensation of heat rising up through the chest, face, and head, followed by flushing and perspiration. Up to 80% of women will experience hot flashes as they go through menopause.[41]

Odai and colleagues[42] evaluated 262 women ages 40 to 65 to determine if there was a relationship between the severity of their hot flashes and any major nutrient. When 43 nutrients were evaluated, only vitamin B6 was found to correlate to the severity of hot flash symptoms. They were further able to find a significant inverse relationship to the consumption of oily fish as the source of vitamin B6 and hot flash severity. Odai and colleagues[42] subsequently recommended consideration of

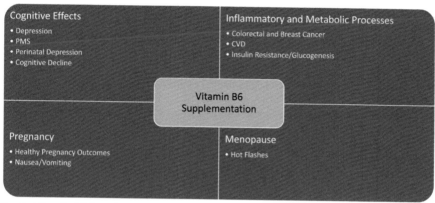

Fig. 1. Vitamin B6 Supplementation.

vitamin B6 and oily fish intake for the reduction of hot flash symptoms caused by the menopausal transition.

SUMMARY

Vitamin B6 or pyroxidine is a crucial nutrient in the body. Serving as a cofactor in over 140 to 150 biochemical reactions in the cell, vitamin B6 plays a vital role in cellular metabolism and physiology.[1,2] Amino acid, glucose, and lipid metabolism and heme and neurotransmitter biosynthesis are among the important reactions that require vitamin B6.[1,2]

Vitamin B6 must be consumed by the body from external sources. With a balanced healthy diet, deficiency is thought to be rare.[2] Yet there are certain medications, health conditions, and dietary weaknesses that predispose to vitamin B6 deficiency.[1] With the water-soluble vitamin B6 levels tightly regulated by the liver, supplementation beyond sufficient is not thought to be beneficial.[5] However, if deficiency does exist, potential sequelae may be severe and detrimental. Overdosage has been shown to be difficult to achieve and only found to occur in extreme mega-doses over longer periods of time. Supplementation with 100 mg daily has been demonstrated to be safe overall and beneficial to anyone with a known or undetected deficiency.[1]

There are various health issues that have particular implications for women. Some are conditions with unique implications for women, while others are specific only to women.[6] Because of the vast array of reactions vitamin B6 is known to facilitate, it is not surprising that vitamin B6 has been found to improve symptoms related to various health issues affecting women. Studies into the cognitive effects of vitamin B6 have shown correlation in symptoms of depression, anxiety, stress,[8,9] premenstrual syndrome,[12–14] perinatal depression,[15] and cognitive decline[4] to either vitamin B6 supplementation or deficiency. Through the vitamin's anti-inflammatory and antioxidant capacities, studies have targeted the vitamin's role in the prevention of breast cancer[3,23] and colorectal cancer,[5,24] finding that vitamin B6 may play an important role in reducing the risk of both. The same inflammatory and immune pathways also lead to the evidence that supports a correlation between vitamin B6 and the reduction of CVD and insulin resistance, with implications for diabetes and lipid dysfunction.[25] Adequate vitamin B6 levels have also been implicated as providing support for healthy pregnancy outcomes,[29] while it plays a well-established role in the management of nausea and vomiting in pregnancy.[38] ACOG[38] recommends vitamin B6 as first-line therapy in the treatment of nausea in pregnancy. Finally, recent evidence suggests an inverse correlation between the severity of hot flashes and vitamin B6 levels.[42]

Although supplementation with vitamin B6 may not be beneficial to those with sufficient vitamin B6 levels,[5] deficiencies may exist in many people because of illness, medications, or nutritional deficits. Vitamin B6 overdosage is only seen in profoundly high doses over long periods of time. Given the data suggesting the prevention of many women's health issues, a supplemental dose of 100 mg daily is unlikely to cause any ill effects, while the potential for benefit exists.[1] **(Fig. 1)**

CLINICS CARE POINTS

- Vitamin B6 deficiency if present results in various ill health effects.
- Supplementation of Vitamin B6 beyond sufficient is not likely useful.
- Correction of Vitamin B6 deficiency is useful.
- Overdose of vitamin B6 is difficult and only seen in extremely high doses over long periods.
- Supplemental vitamin B6 doses of 100 mg daily are considered safe.
- Vitamin B6 supplementation may be helpful in cognitive function disorders, inflammatory and immune conditions, pregnancy outcomes, nausea/vomiting in pregnancy, and hot flashes of menopause.

DISCLOSURE

The author has nothing to disclose.

REFERENCES

1. Parra M, Stahl S, Hellmann H. Vitamin B6 and its role in cell metabolism and physiology. Cells 2018;7(7):84.
2. Ueland M, McCann A, Midttun O, et al. Inflammation, vitamin B6 and related pathways. Mol Aspects Med 2017;53:10-27. https://doi.org/10.1016/j.mam.2016.08.001.
3. Agnoli C, Grioni S, Krogh V, et al. Plasma riboflavin and vitamin B-6, but not homocysteine, folate, or vitamin B-12, are inversely associated with breast cancer risk in the european prospective investigation into cancer and nutrition-varese cohort. J Nutr 2016;146(6):1227–34. Available at: https://www.ncbi.nlm.nih.gov/pubmed/27121532.
4. Palacios N, Scott T, Sahasrabudhe N, et al. Lower plasma vitamin B-6 is associated with 2-year cognitive decline in the Boston Puerto Rican health study. J Nutr 2019;149(4):635–41.
5. Gylling B, Myte R, Schneede J, et al. Vitamin B-6 and colorectal cancer risk: a prospective population-based study using 3 distinct plasma markers of vitamin B-6 status. Am J Clin Nutr 2017;105(4):897–904.
6. National Institutes of Health. Women's health issues. 2020. Available at: https://medlineplus.gov/womenshealth.html. Accessed May 6, 2020.
7. National Institutes of Mental Health. Depression in women: 5 things you should know. 2020. Available at: https://www.nimh.nih.gov/health/publications/depression-in-women/index.shtml. Accessed May 6, 2020.

8. Arévalo SP, Scott TM, Falcón LM, et al. Vitamin B-6 and depressive symptom-atology, over time, in older latino adults. Nutr Neurosci 2019;22(9):625–36.
9. Pouteau E, Kabir-Ahmadi M, Noah L, et al. Superiority of magnesium and vitamin B6 over magnesium alone on severe stress in healthy adults with low magnese-mia: a randomized, single-blind clinical trial. PloS one 2018;13(12):e0208454.
10. Masoumi SZ, Ataollahi M, Oshvandi K. Effect of combined use of calcium and vitamin B6 on premenstrual syndrome symptoms: a randomized clinical trial. J Caring Sci 2016;5(1):67–73.
11. Retallick-Brown H, Blampied N, Rucklidge JJ. A pilot randomized treatment-controlled trial comparing vitamin B6 with broad-spectrum micronutrients for pre-menstrual syndrome. J Altern Complement Med 2020;26(2):88–97.
12. Kashanian M, Mazinani R, Jalalmanesh S. Pyridoxine (vitamin B6) therapy for pre-menstrual syndrome. Int J Gynaecol Obstet 2007;96(1):43–4.
13. Chou P, Morse C, Hong X. A controlled trial of Chinese herbal medicine for pre-menstrual syndrome. J Psychosom Obstet Gynaecol 2008;29(3):189–96.
14. Panay N. Management of premenstrual syndrome: green-top guideline no. 48. BJOG 2009;124(3):e73–105.
15. Khodadad M, Kheirabadi G, Bahadoran P. View of efficacy of vitamin B6 on preg-nancy outcomes. A randomized clinical trial. Journal of Pharmaceutical Research International 2017. https://doi.org/10.9734/JPRI/2017/32675.
16. Shibata K, Tachiki A, Mukaeda K, et al. Changes in plasma pyridoxal 5-phos-phate concentration during pregnancy stages in japanese women. J Nutr Sci Vi-taminol 2013;59(4):343–6.
17. Alzheimer's Association. Women and Alzheimer's. 2020. Available at: https://www.alz.org/alzheimers-dementia/what-is-alzheimers/women-and-alzheimer-s#Quick%20Facts. Accessed May 12, 2020.
18. Tucker KL, Qiao N, Scott T, et al. Highhomocysteine and low B vitamins predict cognitive decline in aging men: the veterans affairs normative aging study. Am J Clin Nutr 2005;82(3):627–35.
19. Hughes C, Ward M, Tracey F, et al. B-vitamin intake and biomarker status in rela-tion to cognitive decline in healthy older adults in a 4-year follow-up study. Nutri-ents 2017;9(53):1–14.
20. Zhang P, Suda T, Suidasari S, et al. Chapter 15 - novel preventive mechanisms of vitamin B6 against inflammation, inflammasome, and chronic diseases. In: Molec-ular nutrition. London: Academic Press, Elsevier; 2020. p. 283–99. https://doi.org/10.1016/B978-0-12-811907-5.00032-4.
21. National Breast Cancer Foundation, Inc. Breast cancer facts. 2019. Available at: https://www.nationalbreastcancer.org/breast-cancer-facts. Accessed May 13, 2020.
22. Roland J, Chun C. What to expect from colon cancer in women 2019. Available at: https://www.jstor.org/stable/23274580.
23. Lurie G, Wilkens LR, Shvetsov YB, et al. Prediagnostic plasma pyridoxal 5'-phos-phate (vitamin B6) levels and invasive breast carcinoma risk: the multiethnic cohort. Cancer Epidemiol Biomarkers Prev 2012;21(11):1942–8.
24. Jia K, Wang R, Tian J. Vitamin B 6 intake and the risk of colorectal cancer: a meta-analysis of prospective cohort studies. Nutr Cancer 2017;69(5):723–31.
25. Liu Z, Li P, Zhao Z, et al. Vitamin B6 prevents endothelial dysfunction, insulin resistance, and hepatic lipid accumulation in [apoe.sup.-/-] mice fed with high-fat diet. J Diabetes Res 2015;2015. https://doi.org/10.1155/2016/1748065.

26. Centers for Disease Control and Prevention. Women and heart disease. 2020. Available at: https://www.cdc.gov/heartdisease/women.htm. Accessed May 6, 2020.

27. National Institute of Diabetes and Digestive and Kidney Diseases. Insulin resistance and prediabetes. 2018. Available at: https://search.credoreference.com/content/entry/ogieamds/insulin_resistance_and_prediabetes/0. Accessed May 13, 2020.

28. Centers for Disease Control and Prevention. Diabetes and women. Diabetes. 2018. Available at: https://www.cdc.gov/diabetes/library/features/diabetes-and-women.html. Accessed May 13, 2020.

29. Ho C, Quay TAW, Devlin AM, et al. Prevalence and predictors of low vitamin B6 status in healthy young adult women in metro Vancouver. Nutrients 2016;8(9):538.

30. US Department of Health and Human Services. Pregnancy complications. 2019. Available at: https://www.womenshealth.gov/pregnancy/youre-pregnant-now-what/pregnancy-complications. Accessed May 6, 2020.

31. Dror DK, Allen LH. Interventions with vitamins B6, B12 and C in pregnancy. Paediatr Perinat Epidemiol 2012;26:55–74.

32. Wachstein M, Graffeo LW. Influence of vitamin B6 on the incidence of preeclampsia. Obstet Gynecol 1956;8:177–80.

33. Roepke JL, Kirksey A. Vitamin B6 nutriture during pregnancy and lactation. Am J Clin Nutr 1969;32:2249–56.

34. Schuster K, Bailey LB, Mahan CS. Vitamin B6 status of low-income adolescent and adult pregnant women and the condition of their infants at birth. Am J Clin Nutr 1981;34:1731–5.

35. Ronnenberg AG, Goldman MB, Chen D, et al. Preconception folate and vitamin B(6) status and clinical spontaneous abortion in Chinese women. Obstet Gynecol 2002;100:107–13.

36. Sharifzadeh F, Kashanian M, Koohpayehzadeh J, et al. A comparison between the effects of ginger, pyridoxine (vitamin B6) and placebo for the treatment of the first trimester nausea and vomiting of pregnancy (NVP). J Matern Fetal Neonatal Med 2018;31(19):2509–14.

37. McParlin C, O'Donnell A, Robson SC, et al. Treatments for hyperemesis gravidarum and nausea and vomiting in pregnancy: a systematic review. JAMA 2016; 316(13):1392–401.

38. American College of Obstetricians and Gynecologists. ACOG practice bulletin no. 189: nausea and vomiting of pregnancy. Obstet Gynecol 2018;131(1): e15–30.

39. Festin M. Nausea and vomiting in early pregnancy. BMJ Clin Evid 2014;2014: 1405.

40. National Institute on Aging. What is menopause. Nurs Stand 2017;30(12):17.

41. Ferrari N. Menopause-related hot flashes and night sweats can last for years. 2015. Available at: https://www.health.harvard.edu/blog/menopause-related-hot-flashes-night-sweats-can-last-years-201502237745. Accessed May 18, 2020.

42. Odai T, Terauchi M, Hirose A, et al. Severity of hot flushes is inversely associated with dietary intake of vitamin B6 and oily fish. Climacteric 2019;22(6):617–21. Available at: http://www.tandfonline.com/doi/abs/10.1080/13697137.2019. 1609440.

Fat-Soluble Vitamins

Sherri L. Stevens, PhD, RN

KEYWORDS

- Fat-soluble vitamins • Vitamins • Nutrition

KEY POINTS

- Fat-soluble vitamins A, D, E, and K are obtained in a well-balanced diet.
- The fat-soluble vitamins are stored in the body and are involved with many body systems to maintain homeostasis.
- Individuals with chronic health diseases may have low levels of required fat-soluble vitamins.

INTRODUCTION

Vitamins are necessary micronutrients required by the human body for growth and development. Vitamins are obtained through diets. Vitamins can be classified as water soluble and fat soluble. Water-soluble vitamins are consumed in the diet but the excesses are excreted from the body. Fat-soluble vitamins are stored in the body in fatty tissues and the liver.

The fat-soluble vitamin are vitamins A, D, E, and K. Each of the fat-soluble vitamins is divided further into other groups, depending on molecular structure. Vitamin A is classified into 2 forms. One form consists of the retinoids, which includes retinol, retinal, and the retinyl esters. The other forms of vitamin A are the carotenoids. Carotenoids, such as beta carotene, are plant sources converted into vitamin A.[1,2] Vitamin E is classified into tocopherols, containing 4 subgroups, and the tocotrienols, also consisting of 4 subgroups.[3] Vitamin K is classified into the phylloquinones and menaquinones. Finally, vitamin D is classified into vitamin D_2 ergosterol and vitamin D_3 cholecalciferol.[4] There are complex processes involved with the absorption and metabolism of each of the fat-soluble vitamins once they enter the body. Fat-soluble vitamins are absorbed in the intestines requiring a series of metabolic processes and the presence of fat.[5] Each of the fat-soluble vitamins contains unique structures and must be transported into the circulation with carrier proteins or lipoproteins.[6] The vitamins then are transported to the liver or other adipose tissue for use and storage. Deficiencies of the fat-soluble vitamins can have an impact on many systems in the body, especially the immune system. The fat-soluble vitamins have strong roles in

School of Nursing, Middle Tennessee State University, MTSU Box 81, Murfreesboro, TN 37132, USA
E-mail address: Sherri.Stevens@mtsu.edu

the immune system and deficiencies can have an impact on overall health and well-being.[7,8]

There are standards of measurements used by nutritional and government agencies, such as the Food and Nutrition Board of the Institute of Medicine of the National Academy of Sciences and the National Institutes of Health (NIH), to provide the guidelines for adequate amounts of fat-soluble vitamins required per day.[9,10] The US Food and Drug Administration (FDA) determines the daily values for all food nutrients.[11] The FDA has 2 distinguished groups for measurement; 1 is the daily reference value for carbohydrates, fats, and proteins and the other is the reference daily intakes for vitamins and minerals (Food and Nutrition Board of the Institute of Medicine, National Academy of Sciences, 2020). The estimated average requirements are measured by the average daily nutrient intake level that is estimated to meet the requirements of half of the healthy adults in a group. The recommended dietary allowance is measured as the daily dietary intake level needed to meet the nutrient requirements of up to 98% of healthy individuals in a group and the tolerable upper limit measurement is the maximum adult daily intake unlikely to cause harm to the individual (NIH). Vitamin amounts may be identified in different ways on food labels, depending on what measurement standard was used.

Those at risk of fat-soluble vitamin deficiencies include the elderly and patients with diagnosed malabsorption issues.[1,12,13] Due to the aging process, the immune system in the elderly is not as effective at responding and fighting infections. The elderly also may suffer from poor nutritional intake, which can have an impact on health.[1,2] An analysis of each of the fat-soluble vitamins is presented to outline the unique contribution of each to maintain homeostasis.

HISTORY OF VITAMIN A

The symptoms of vitamin A deficiency have been documented for more than 3000 years in many different cultures. The symptoms of poor vision, blindness, and corneal changes have been described and recorded with ancient treatments and home remedies. Night blindness symptoms and treatments were found documented in the Egyptian Ebers Papyrus, 1500 BC[14] According to Egyptian history, it was recommended to apply roasted ox liver to the eyes. The Greeks recorded eating raw beef liver soaked in honey to improve night vision.[15] Today it is known that most of the body's vitamin A is stored in the liver.

In the 1800s, a French physician, Bitot would identify and record details of white spots on the cornea of people with night blindness, which eventually would be called Bitot spots. The diagnosis of the Bitot spots is affiliated with vitamin A deficiencies.[16] These spots contain keratinized epithelium cells and gram-negative rods. In 1913, vitamin A was discovered by Elmer McCollum, a biochemist who constantly studied human and animal nutrition.[17] From 1913 through 1922, McCollum and others would identify and discover vitamins A, B, D, and E while working with animals, diets, and nutrition.

DISCUSSION OF VITAMIN A

The molecular structure of vitamin A consists of a complex structure with 20 carbon structures, a Methycyclohexane ring, a hydroxyl group (retinol), an aldehyde group (retinal), and a carboxylic acid group (retinoic acid).[9] It is described as a yellow fat-soluble antioxidant vitamin. Vitamin A has different forms, including preformed vitamin A from animal sources retinol, retinoic acid, and retinal, which are considered as the retinoids. There also are provitamin A compounds, such as the carotenoids lycopene, lutein, and beta carotene, obtained from plant sources.[18] These nutrients also must be obtained in the diet. During digestion, vitamin A is absorbed in the intestines through a process involving the enterocytes before entering the lymphatic circulation.[5] Vitamin A has a role in vision, the growth and development of the cells of the embryo, the immune system, and the support of epithelial cells. It also is considered an important antioxidant that contributes to multiple health purposes.[19] There are hepatic stellate cells located in the liver that store up to 80% of vitamin A in the form of retinyl palmitate, which is present in lipid droplets and available to supply the body.[20]

Vitamin A has a role in maintaining the lining of epithelial cells in the mucosa.[8] The epithelial cells provide a barrier support throughout the body, which provides protection against microorganisms. Conditions, such as diarrhea, can disrupt the mucosal lining in the gastrointestinal tract and may create a deficiency of vitamin A due to malabsorption.

Retinol is hydrolyzed in the intestines before it can be absorbed by the enterocytes. While in the enterocytes, the retinol components are turned into chylomicrons and can be distributed to the circulation and into the tissues.

Vitamin A has an impact on the immune system. It is involved with the innate and cell-mediated immunity and the humoral antibody response.[8] The innate immune system includes barriers such as the skin, cellular lining of the gastrointestinal tract and respiratory tract, and secretions, such as tears. The humoral antibody response of the immune system involves antibodies and antigens to protect against various pathogens that may enter the body.[21] Vitamin A has a role in antibodies responding to infections in the body.[2] Retinoic acid assists with the levels of natural killer cells, which can provide antitumor and antiviral activity in the body.[22] Retinoic acid also helps to increase the phagocytic activity in macrophages and increases the interleukin (IL)-1 and other cytokines to serve as mediators of inflammation. It also assists with production of B lymphocytes and T lymphocytes. It has been documented that vitamin A can have an impact on the body's reaction and defense against the measles virus due to its impact on the immune system.[2] The World Health Organization (WHO) recommends oral doses of vitamin A for 2 days for children over the age of 1 who have the measles in countries known to have vitamin A deficiencies, such as some countries in Africa.[23]

Vitamin A eye drops or ointment may be used to prevent dry eyes. Vitamin A eye drops also may be used for those patients in the intensive care unit who may have impaired ocular responses.[24,25] Some studies have found that application of a topical form of vitamin A in the eyes can assist with the production of corneal epithelial cells, improve epithelial cell damage, and provide moisture to the eye for comfort.[26]

Vitamin A can be used for a variety of skin conditions to promote healing. Vitamin A can be used for wound healing to stimulate the growth of cells. It also restores the epithelial structure of wounds contributing to healing. Products, such as hydrogel with alginate, vitamins A and E, and fatty acids, can be used for wound healing as well.[27] The alginate products along with vitamins A, E, and fatty acids can promote the formation of collagen in a wound to enhance the healing process.[28]

Vitamin A products can be used to treat dermatology lesions, acne, and psoriasis. For example, topical retinoic acid medications may be used to treat acne. The effects on the epidermal cells result in reducing inflammation of the skin. Antibiotics also may be used along with retinoid products to reduce areas of inflammation. A stronger vitamin A product used for treating acne is isotretinoin (or Accutane®), which may cause extreme drying of the face and lips during treatment. High doses of vitamin A can cause birth defects; thus, pregnant women should not take this product. This medication requires strict health care management between the patient and the provider.[29]

Topical vitamin A products, such as tretinoin, may be used to reduce wrinkles or mottled dark spots on the face. This product may cause exfoliation and redness during treatment. Other products, such as retinol, a topical form of vitamin A, contributes to the skin by encouraging hydration of the cells and is available in many skin care anti-aging products.[30]

DEFICIENCIES OF VITAMIN A

Xerophthalmia and night blindness can result from vitamin A deficiency.[12,31] Drying of the conjunctiva and increasing opacity of the cornea occurs with the lack of vitamin A to protect the eye structure. In 2009, the WHO reported night blindness in more than 19 million pregnant women and 190 million children due to vitamin A deficiency. Guidelines were established to provide vitamin A supplementation to prevent blindness. According to the WHO, vitamin A supplementation has been provided to children in many regions, such as Africa and South East Asia, where deficiency of this vitamin has been identified as a health problem. Some countries have established fortifying foods, such as wheat flour, corn meal, and rice, with vitamin A as well to improve health.[32]

Conditions resulting from vitamin A deficiency can cause dryness of epithelial cells in the gastrointestinal tract, respiratory tract, and genitourinary tract. Dryness and irritation decrease the ability of the cells to provide protection and ward off infections. The lack of normal redeveloping tissue in mucosal linings in the body due to infection can decrease the function of neutrophils, natural killer cells, and macrophages.[33] Vitamin A deficiencies also may interfere with neutrophil development and cytokine release, which can contribute to increased opportunities of inflammation.[5] Vitamins A deficiency can cause impairment of the immune system by altering the innate and the adaptive immune response that automatically occur tin response to infections.

Most milk in the United States is fortified with vitamin A. Due to the process of making low fat milk, some of the vitamin A is lost; thus, vitamin A may be added as vitamin A–retinol, vitamin A–acetate retinyl, or vitamin A–palmitate–retinyl palmitate (see **Table 1** for Vitamin A food sources).[34,35]

Table 1 Vitamin A		
Vitamin A Requirements	**Function**	**Food Sources**
Adult men, 900 µg RAE	• Vision	Black-eyed peas
Adult women, 700 µg RAE	• Cell growth	Butter
	• Antioxidant	Cantaloupe
	• Skin/wound	Carrots
	• Red blood cell formation	Cheese
		Egg yolk
		Fish liver oils
		Green leafy vegetables
		Kale
		Liver
		Mangoes
		Milk
		Red peppers
		Squash
		Spinach
		Sweet potatoes

Abbreviation: RAE, retinol activity equivalents.
NIH office of dietary supplements, US department of health and human services.

HISTORY OF VITAMIN D

The disease known as rickets has been mentioned in writings since the Roman empire. Soranus of Ephesus, a Greek physician, wrote of infant children trying to sit and stand, with distorted legs.[36] In the 1550s, others described pale children who could not stand. Records from China, Holland, Switzerland, and London all have documented descriptions of the mysterious bone deformities in children. In 1634, in London, the term rickets appeared in the Annual Bill of Mortality of the City of London, a document listing recorded deaths.[36] The condition known as rickets was described as curved bones, deformed bones, and bowed bones in the writings by Daniel Whistler and James Glisson in 1650 in England.[37] Eventually, Elmer Verner McCollum and others would identify a substance, a vitamin involving calcium as a cause for the bone deformities. This vitamin was discovered more than 100 years ago through the work of Funk and McCollum.[38] Conducting research with animals, diet and sunlight experimentation observations were recorded. In the 1930s, the vitamin D structure would be isolated and identified by Askew, and, in 1937, vitamin D_3 would be identified by Windaus.[39]

Vitamin D often is called the sunshine vitamin. Exposure to sunlight allows the vitamin D to be synthesized in the skin.[39] Vitamin D7 also is considered a prohormone.[4] Vitamin D is a fat-soluble vitamin present in foods, such as dairy products, eggs, and fish. Vitamin D is classified further into D7-dehydrocholesterol, also known as vitamin D_3, and vitamin D_2, also known as ergosterol.[40] Vitamin D_2, ergocalciferol, is obtained through food sources and the fortification of food. A form of vitamin D_3 is involved with the absorption of calcium and phosphorus in the intestine, which is eventually used to impact bone mineralization.

DISCUSSION OF VITAMIN D

Vitamin D is responsible for the regulation and distribution of calcium and phosphorus in the body. Vitamin D is associated with growing bones and the skeletal system.[41] Vitamin D is consumed through the diet and from the ultraviolet rays of the sun. It undergoes a unique chemical process in the body that can have an impact on other cells and tissues. The major function of vitamin D is to assist with the serum phosphorus and calcium concentrations required for bone and cells.[42] Vitamin D works in the bone by promoting the productions of osteoblasts and osteoclasts. In the body, vitamin D is located in the bone and assists with osteoclastogenesis. Osteocalcin is a Gla protein produced by the osteoblast cells in the bone. The production of osteocalcin is regulated by vitamin D.

Vitamin D also is present in the parathyroid glands and has a role in parathyroid hormone secretion. In the intestinal area, vitamin D is involved with calcium and phosphorus absorption that is circulated and used and many parts of the body. There are vitamin D receptors located on the immature cells in the thymus gland as well as the mature lymphocytes.[8] Vitamin D also has a role in cellular development.[37] This allows for participation in the immune response. Vitamin D is transported to the liver and eventually to the kidney. In the kidney, vitamin D is involved with renal tissue and the renin angiotensin system.

DEFICIENCIES OF VITAMIN D

A deficiency of vitamin D can result in an interference with mineralization in the bones, resulting in rickets, osteoporosis, and osteomalacia. Vitamin D deficiency affects the growth and strength of bones in children and bone density in adults. Osteomalacia, or softening and demineralization of the bones, occurs in adults resulting in bone pain and increases the risk of osteoporosis.

Low levels of vitamin D are common in the elderly. It is recommended for the elderly to take vitamin D supplements to maintain bone density strength.[12] Hip fractures are common in the elderly population and are associated with osteoporosis. Each year thousands are hospitalized with hip fractures and many are women over the age of 50. According to Combs and McClung,[37] it is estimated that there will be 3 million osteoporosis-related fractures to occur in the United States by 2025 at a cost of $16 billion to $25 billion dollars. A lack of vitamin D can cause decreased absorption of intestinal calcium and phosphorus. Secondary causes of vitamin D deficiency can be related to conditions, such as hypoparathyroidism, hepatitis, and gastrointestinal diseases; all can decrease levels of vitamin D in the body.[37]

Vitamin D fortification in milk began in the 1930s.[43] Fortification is a process of adding food nutrients, such as vitamins, to food to prevent diseases, such as rickets.[44] The development and process of fortification would become a standard of practice endorsed by the American Medical Association Council on Foods and Nutrition.[45] Eventually, vitamin A would be added to some foods, such as milk as well. Vitamin A currently is added to milk in the form of retinyl palmitate (**Table 2**).

HISTORY OF VITAMIN E

Vitamin E is a lipid-soluble component with a molecular structure made from a chromanol ring with a chain. Vitamin E has 2 groups, tocotrienols and tocopherols, and each of these groups is divided further into isomers.[4,46] Vitamin E was first described and discussed regarding the various tocol types in 1922 by Evans and Bishop while working with rat research.[47] In 1935, vitamin E was isolated in its pure form.

DISCUSSION OF VITAMIN E

Vitamin E has been described as an antioxidant with anti-inflammatory properties that may assist with the prevention of atherosclerosis.[48] Vitamin E is described as having an important role in the immune system, because it appears in higher concentrations in the immune cells in comparison to other cells in the body.[49] Alpha-tocopherol has been identified as the primary form of vitamin E in the plasma.

Table 2
Vitamin D

Vitamin D Requirements	Functions	Food Sources
Adult men, ages 51–70 years 600 IU 15 µg Adult men, ages >70 years 800 IU 20 µg Adult women, ages 51–70 years 600 IU 15 µg Adult women ages >70 years 800 IU 20 µg	• Bone development • Production of osteoclastin • Prevention of osteoporosis • Regulate calcium and Phosphorus • Immune response	Cheese Eggs Foods fortified with vitamin D: milk and dairy products, cereals Margarine Mushrooms Salmon Trout

NIH office of dietary supplements, US department of health and human services.

In order for vitamin E to be absorbed, micelles must be formed from pancreatic and biliary secretions. Once micelles are formed, vitamin E can be moved to the intestine. Once in the intestine, chylomicron then is secreted and vitamin E can be moved into the circulation through the lymphatic paths. Vitamin E is delivered to the liver; it returns back into the circulation through lipoproteins. Lipoproteins transport vitamin E in the blood.

As an antioxidant, vitamin E is involved with inhibiting the oxidation process. Oxidation occurs due to a chemical reaction causing the production of free radicals, which can result in damage to cells. Vitamin E has the ability to protect the cells from damage caused by free radicals formed in the body.

Due to the antioxidant activity of vitamin E, it is able to provide cellular membrane integrity. It has a role with the growth of erythrocytes and has been associated with impacting the aging process.[5] Vitamin E also inhibits protein kinase activity, resulting in platelet aggregation, which may decrease atherosclerosis.[3] The antioxidant and anti-inflammatory properties also may have an impact on cardiovascular disease.[48] There have been studies (HOPE and HOPE-TOO) using high doses of vitamin E that failed to support a decreased risk of cardiovascular events in people over the age of 50.[50]

Vitamin E also has a role in suppressing the formation of inflammatory cytokines tumor necrosis factor, IL-1, IL-6, and IL-8 in animal studies.[5] Vitamin E appears to boost the immune system in humans and animals.[3] Vitamin E may be helpful in Alzheimer disease due to the antioxidant properties as well.[51] There are studies, however, with conflicting results regarding vitamin E and Alzheimer disease.

DEFICIENCIES OF VITAMIN E

Individuals diagnosed with malabsorption problems may have vitamin E deficiencies due to the absorption process with pancreatic secretions, bile, and fats.[52] For example, conditions such as chronic hepatitis, fat malabsorption, gastrectomy, pancreatic disorders, and cystic fibrosis. Vitamin E deficiencies also can occur in babies with hemolytic anemia (see **Table 3** for Vitamin E food sources).[53]

Table 3 Vitamin E		
Vitamin E Requirements	**Functions**	**Food Sources**
Adults 15 mg/d UL 100 mg/d	• Antioxidant properties • Immune system • Cell membrane integrity • Red blood cell formation • Prevents platelet aggregation	Almonds Animal fat Asparagus Fish Nuts Olive oil Palm oil Peanuts Peanut butter Plant oils Pumpkin Safflower oil Sunflower oil Sunflower seeds Wheat germ oil

NIH office of dietary supplements, US department of health and human services.

HISTORY OF VITAMIN K

Vitamin K first was discovered in 1929 by Henrik Dam, who would be awarded the Nobel Prize in Medicine for his years of work regarding vitamin K and coagulation.[54] Dam, a biochemist, discovered vitamin K through his work with the diet and metabolism in chickens. Initially, Dam described this vitamin and named it vitamin K after the German pronunciation of *koagulation*, due to the effects of coagulation.[55] Vitamin K would continue to be studied for many years. At room temperature, vitamin K is described as a yellow oil, with some compounds or vitamers described as yellow crystals.[56] The structure consists of 2-methyl-1,4-napthoquinone with a side chain.

DISCUSSION OF VITAMIN K

Vitamin K is produced by plants and obtained through the diet, although some vitamin K is available in the intestines. Vitamin K absorption requires actions of the pancreas, bile, and fat components. Some vitamin K is absorbed by the enterocytes and transported to the liver. Once in the liver, a process occurs whereby vitamin K coagulation proteins can store the vitamin. Vitamin K through complex processes combines with specific proteins. Among the group of proteins are Gla vitamin K–dependent proteins. There are Gla vitamin K proteins in the bone that contribute to bone health (see **Table 4** for Vitamin K food sources).[56]

Vitamin K is associated with several factors in the blood coagulation process. These are prothrombin (or factor II), factor VII, factor IX, and factor X. Vitamin K is required for prothrombin synthesis and for blood coagulation. A deficiency of vitamin K can result in bleeding. Vitamin K was established as a treatment of hemorrhage in a patient with obstructive jaundice and prothrombin clotting deficiency in 1938.[57]

Babies are born without vitamin K and are required to receive a prophylaxis vitamin K injection to stimulate prothrombin levels. Typically, newborns receive a vitamin K injection shortly after birth. The American Academy of Pediatrics standard for the United States is 1 mg of vitamin K for newborns.[58] Over the past few years, there has been an increased resistance to prophylactic immunizations, including the vitamin K injection. There have been some parents refusing the vitamin K injection to be given.[59] A study performed in Tennessee (2013) to survey parents' refusal of vitamin K injections found 31% of infants born in birthing centers did not receive the prophylactic injection.[60]

Vitamin K antagonists, such as warfarin, were developed in the 1940s. Warfarin acts in the body by slowing the production of certain clotting mechanisms and this interaction

Table 4 Vitamin K		
Vitamin K Requirements	**Functions**	**Food Sources**

Measured by adequate intake Adult men, 120 µg Adult women, 90 µg	• Blood clotting
	• Blood coagulation factors
	  ○ Prothrombin factor II
	  ○ Factor VII
	  ○ Factor IX
	  ○ Factor X
	• Gla K proteins for bone mineralization
		Dark green vegetables Asparagus Beef Broccoli Brusssels sprouts Cabbage Eggs Fish Liver Peas Spinach

NIH office of dietary supplements, US department of health and human services.

produces a deficiency of vitamin K. In the event of a warfarin overdose, injectable vitamin K can be administered to reverse the effects of hypoprothrombinemia and bleeding. Injectable vitamin K has a brand names of AquaMEPHYTON (PHYTONADIPNE, Teligent Pharma), Phylloquinone, and Mephyton and a generic name of phytonadione.[61]

DEFICIENCIES OF VITAMIN K

Vitamin K deficiency is observed with coagulopathy signs, such as prolonged clotting time and subcutaneous bleeding. Low vitamin K levels also may contribute to poor bone density in some people due to the vitamin K Gla proteins' involvement with bone structure and mineralization. Vitamin K levels that are deficient may be identified with osteoporosis.[56]

Vitamin K deficiency appears to be a factor in chronic kidney disease patients and could be related to the diet. Diets consisting of low potassium and low phosphate intake may contribute to low vitamin K requirements. Vitamin K is required for Gla protein production, which prevents tissue calcification.[62] Tissue calcification can cause deposits to build up in the vessels leading to vascular calcification, which has an impact on the cardiovascular status of the kidney patient. Patients receiving hemodialysis via arteriovenous fistula are at risk for calcification and thrombosis of the site. These patients may be prescribed anticoagulation medications, which are vitamin K antagonists and may contribute to vitamin K deficiency.

Anticoagulant medications, also known as vitamin K antagonists, contribute to vitamin K deficiency. Medications, such as warfarin and salicylates, can decrease vitamin K levels in the body. Low levels of vitamin K in the body can be identified by prolonged clotting time. Medications, such as cephalosporins and broad-spectrum antibiotics, may decrease vitamin K production in gastrointestinal bacteria.

Hemorrhagic disease that occurs in some newborns was detailed by Charles Townsend in 1894.[63] Townsend described bleeding problems that occurred to newborn babies 2 to 3 days of being born. Vitamin K deficiency bleeding is due to low vitamin K levels in the newborn, which creates low vitamin K clotting factors. This can result in hemorrhages of the skin and gastrointestinal tract and intracranial hemorrhage. The symptoms of bleeding can occur during the first 24 hours up to a late onset occurring 12 weeks after birth.[64] The complications of bleeding in the newborn can be prevented by administering the synthetic vitamin K injection after birth.

SUMMARY

Fat-soluble vitamins are involved with many physiologic processes in the body. The fat-soluble vitamins have a complex absorption process requiring involvement of the pancreas, bile enzymes, and fats. Once in the body, these vitamins are absorbed and stored for future use. A well-balanced diet provides the necessary requirements of the fat-soluble vitamins. Vitamins A, D, E, and K are closely involved with the immune system and the protection of the cells. These vitamins also are linked to wound healing, cellular integrity, the cardiovascular system, the renal system, the endocrine system, bone health, and the aging process. Further research is needed to identify the power of these vitamins in a compromised patient.

CLINICS CARE POINTS

- Fat soluble vitamins are absorbed through complex mechanisms in the digestive system and stored in the body for future use.
- Fat soluble vitamins have unique characteristics that impact the immune system.

- Deficiencies of fat soluble vitamins can impact overall health and the strength of the immune system in combating illness.

DISCLOSURE

The author has nothing to disclose.

REFERENCES

1. Thomas DR. Vitamins in aging, health, and longevity. Clin Interv Aging 2006;1(1): 81–91.
2. Riccioni G, D'Orazio N, Menna V, et al. Fat soluble vitamins and immune system: an overview. Eur J Inflamm 2003;1(2):59–64.
3. Lee GY, Han SN. The role of Vitamin E in immunity. Nutrients 2018;10(11):161.
4. Borel P, Desmarchelier C. Bioavailability of fat-soluble vitamins and phytochemicals in humans: effects of genetic variation. Annu Rev Nutr 2018;38:69–96.
5. Albahrani AA, Greaves RF. Fat-soluble vitamins: clinical indications and current challenges for chromatographic measurement. Clin Biochem Rev 2016;37(1): 27–47.
6. Kono N, Arai H. Intracellular transport of fat-soluble vitamins A and E. Traffic 2015;16(1):19–34.
7. Maggini S, Pierre A, Calder PC. Review immune and micronutrient requirements change over the life course. Nutrients 2018;10:1531.
8. Alpert PT. The role of vitamins and minerals on the immune system. Home Health Care Manag Pract 2017;29:199–202.
9. Institute of Medicine. Dietary Reference Intakes: The Essential Guide to Nutrient Requirements. Washington, DC: The National Academies Press; 2006. https://doi.org/10.17226/11537.
10. US Department of Health and Human Services. National health institute: office of dietary supplements. Nutrient recommendations: dietary reference intakes (DRI). Available at: https://ods.od.nih.gov/Health_Information/Dietary_Reference_Intakes.aspx#:%7E:text=%2C%20National%20Academy%20of%20Sciences.,intake%2C%20nutrition%2C%20and%20health. Accessed June 15, 2020.
11. US Food & Drug Administration. Interactive nutrition facts label. What's new with the nutrition facts label. 2020. Available at: https://www.fda.gov/food/new-nutrition-facts-label/whats-new-nutrition-facts-label. Accessed June 14, 2020.
12. Csapo J, Albert Cs, Prokisch J. The role of vitamins in the diet of the elderly I. Fat-soluble vitamins. Acta Universitatis Sapientiae, Alimentaria 2017;10:127–45.
13. DiBaise M, Tarelto SM. Hair, nails, and skin: differentiating cutaneous manifestations of micronutrient deficiency. Nutr Clin Pract 2019;34(4):490–503.
14. Ebell B. The greatest egyptian medical document. Copenhagen (Denmark): Munksgaard and Oxford University Press; 1937. The Papyrus Ebers.
15. Hajar AH, Binali Al. Night blindness and ancient remedy. Heart Views 2014;15(4): 136–9.
16. Wolf G. Milestones in biological Research. A history of Vitamin A and retinoids. FASEB J 1996;10(9):1102–7.
17. Semba RD. On the 'discovery' of vitamin A. Ann Nutr Metab 2012;61(3):192–8.
18. Mozos I, Stoian D, Luca CT. Crosstalk between Vitamins A, B12, D, K, C, and E status and arteria stiffness. Dis Markers 2017;2017:8784971.
19. Ashor AW, Siervo M, Lara J, et al. Antioxidant vitamin supplementation reduces arterial stiffness in adults: a systematic review and meta-analysis of randomized controlled trials. J Nutr 2014;144(10):1594–602.

20. Senoo H, Mezaki Y, Fujiwara M. The stellate cell system (vitamin A-storing cell system). Anat Sci Int 2017;92(4):387–455.
21. Castelo-Branco C, Soveral I. The immune system and aging: a review. Gynecol Endocrinol 2014;30:16–22.
22. Zhao Z, Ross AC. Retinoic acid repletion restores the number of leukocytes and their subsets and stimulates natural cytotoxicity in vitamin A-deficient rats. J Nutr 1995;125(8):p2064–73.
23. World Health Organization. Food and agricultural organization of the united nations. Global prevalence of vitamin A deficiency in populations at risk 1995-2005 WHO global database on Vitamin A deficiency 2009. Available at: https://www.who.int/nutrition/publications/micronutrients/vitamin_a_deficiency/9789241598019/en/. Accessed June 15, 2020.
24. Babamohamadi H, Nobahar M, Razi J. Comparing Vitamin A and moist chamber in preventing ocular surface disorders. Clin Nurs Res 2018;27(6):714–29.
25. Selek H, Unlu N, Orhan M, et al. Evaluation of retinoic acid ophthalmic emulsion in dry eye. Eur J Ophthalmol 2000;10(2):121–7.
26. Hori Y, Spurr-Michaud SJ, Russo CL, et al. Effect of retinoic acid on gene expression in human conjunctival epithelium: secretory phospholipase A2 mediates retinoic acid induction of MUC16. Invest Ophthalmol Vis Sci 2005;46(11):4050–61.
27. Rosa CA, Paggiaro AO, Fernandes de Carvalho V. Effect of hydrogel enriched with Alginate, fatt acids, and vitamins A and E on pressure injuries: a case series. Plast Surg Nurs 2019;39(3):87–94.
28. Summa M, Russo D, Penna I, et al. A biocompatible sodium alginate/povidone iodine film enhances wound healing. Eur J Pharm Biopharm 2018;122:17–24.
29. Burchum JR, Rosenthal LD. Drugs for the skin. In: Lehne's pharmacology for nursing care. 2019. 10th edition. St Louis (MO): Elsevier; 2019. p. 1284–91.
30. Hodulik G. Skin hydration 2016. p. 33–7. Available at: http://www.SkinInc.com. Accessed June 14,2020.
31. Tanumihardjo SA, Russell RM, Stephensen CB, et al. Biomarkers of nutrition for development (BOND)—vitamin A review. J Nutr 2016;146(9):1816S–48S.
32. World Health Organization. Global nutrition policy review 2016-2017: country progress in creating enabling policy environments for promoting healthy diets and nutrition 2018. Available at: https://www.who.int/publications/i/item/9789241514873. Accessed June 15, 2020.
33. Stephenson CB. Vitamin A, infection, and immune function. Annu Rev Nutr 2001;21:167–92.
34. The dairy practices council (July, 2001). Guidelines for Vitamin A & D fortification of fluid milk. Available at: https://phpa.health.maryland.gov/OEHFP/OFPCHS/Milk/Shared%20Documents/DPC053_Vitamin_AD_Fortification_Fluid_Milk.pdf. Accessed June 12, 2020.
35. Centers for disease control and prevention (CDC). Nutrition. Fortified Cow's milk and milk alternatives. 2020. Available at: https://www.cdc.gov/nutrition/infantandtoddlernutrition/foods-and-drinks/cows-milk-and-milk-alternatives.html. Accessed June 15, 2020.
36. O'Riordan LHJ, Bijvoet OLM. Rickets before the discovery of Vitamin D. Bonekey Rep 2014;3:478.
37. Combs GF, McClung JP. Chapter 7 Vitamin D. In: The Vitamins fundamental aspects in nutrition and health. 5th edition. Westborough (MA): Elsevier; 2017. p. 161–206.
38. Wintermeyer E, Ihl C, Ehnert S, et al. Crucial role of Vitamin D in the musculoskeletal system. Nutrients 2016;8:319.

39. DeLuca HF. History of the discovery of vitamin D and its active metabolites. Bonekey Rep 2014;3:479.
40. Kraemer K, Semba RD, Eggersdorfer M. Introduction: the diverse and essential biological functions of vitamins. Ann Nutr Metab 2012;61(3):185–91.
41. Aranow C. Vitamin D and the immune system. J Investig Med 2011;59(6):881–6.
42. Eisman JA, Bouillon R. Vitamin D: direct effects of vitamin D metabolites on bone: lessons from genetically modified mice. Bonekey Rep 2014;3:499.
43. Yeh EB, Barbano DM, Drake M. Vitamin fortification of fluid milk. J Food Sci 2017; 82(4):856–64.
44. Alvarez VB. Fluid milk and cream products. The sensory evaluation of diary products. USA: Springer; 2009. p. 73–133.
45. Stevenson EH. Importance of vitamin D milk. American Medical Association Council Foods Nutrition 1955;159:1018–9.
46. Traber MG. Vitamin E regulatory mechanisms. Annu Rev Nutr 2007;27:347–62.
47. Traber M, Sies H. Vitamin E in humans: demand and delivery. Annu Rev Nutr 1996;16:321–47.
48. Singh U, Devaraj S, Jialal I. Vitamin E, oxidative stress, and inflammation. Annu Rev Nutr 2005;25:151–74.
49. Lewis ED, Meydani SN, Wu D. Regulatory role of vitamin E in the immune system and inflammation. IUBMB Life 2019;71(4):487–94.
50. Lonn E, Yusuf S, Hoogwerf B, et al, MICRO-HOPE Study. Effects of Vitamin E on cardiovascular and microvascular outcomes in high-risk patients with diabetes: results of the HOPE Study and MICRO-HOPE substudy. Diabetes Care 2002; 25(11):1919–27.
51. Grimm MOW, Mett J, Hartmann T. The impact of Vitamin E and other fat-soluble vitamins on Alzheimer's disease. Int J Mol Sci 2016;17(11):1785.
52. Traber MG. Vitamin E- Alpha-tocopherol. In: Herrmann W, Obeid R, editors. Vitamins in the prevention of human disease. Berlin (Germany): Walter de Gruyter; 2011. p. P457–82.
53. Koletzko B, Decsi T, Sawatzki G. Vitamin E status of low birthweight infants fed formula enriched with long-chain polyunsaturated fatty acids. Int J Vitam Nutr Res 1995;65(2):101–4.
54. Ferland G. Vitamin K, an emerging nutrient in brain function. Biofactors 2012; 38(2):151–7.
55. Dam H. The antihaemorrhagic vitamin of the chick. Biochem J 1935;29(6): 1273–85.
56. Combs GF, McClung JP. Chapter 9 Vitamin K. In: The vitamins fundamental aspects in nutrition and health. 5th edition. Westborough (MA): Elsevier; 2017. p. 243–65.
57. Smith HP, Warner ED, Brinkhous KM, et al. Bleeding tendency and prothrombin deficiency in biliary fistula dogs: effect of feeding bile And Vitamin K. J Exp Med 1938;67(6):911–20.
58. American Academy of Pediatrics Committee on Fetus and Newborn. Controversies concerning Vitamin K and the newborn. Pediatrics 2003;112(1 Pt 1): 191–2.
59. Loyal J, Taylor JA, Phillipi CA, et al. Refusal of Vitamin K by parents of newborns: a survey of the better outcomes through research for newborns network. Acad Pediatr 2017;17(4):368–73.
60. Marcewicz LH, Clayton J, Maenner M, et al. Parental refusal of Vitamin K and neonatal preventive services: a need for surveillance. Matern Child Health J 2017;21(5):1079–84.

61. Lippi G, Franchini M. Vitamin K in neonates: facts and myths. Blood Transfus 2011;9(1):4–9.
62. Cozzolino M, Mangano M, Galassi A, et al. Vitamin K in chronic kidney disease. Nutrients 2019;11(1):168.
63. Mihatsch WA, Braegger C, Bronsky J, et al. ESPGHAN committee on nutrition. Prevention of vitamin K deficiency bleeding in newborn infants: a position paper by the ESPGHAN committee on nutrition. J Pediatr Gastroenterol Nutr 2016;63(1): 123–9.
64. Johnson PJ. Vitamin K prophylaxis in the newborn: indications and controversies. Neonatal Netw 2013;32(3):193–9.

Vitamin D: Vitamin or Hormone?

Deborah L. Ellison, PhD, MSN, BSN*,
Heather R. Moran, MSN, BSN, CRRN, CMSRN

KEYWORDS

- Vitamin D • Vitamin D and pain • Pathophysiology of vitamin D
- Vitamin D as a hormone • Uses of vitamin D

KEY POINTS

- The early application of vitamin D as a key skeletal element has been augmented more recently by apparent extra-skeletal effects of vitamin D.
- The most common form, cholecalciferol, or vitamin D_3, is synthesized in the skin after exposure to ultraviolet B radiation or sunlight.
- Additionally, calcitriol has been shown to have enhancing effects on the cardiac systems, the endocrine system, the immune system, and other metabolic pathways.
- Almost all cells and tissues in the body are now recognized as having VDRs, which is why it can be linked to other various systems and diseases.

INTRODUCTION

The essential role of vitamin D in bone health has been known for more than a century.

According to existing literature, vitamin D deficiency is a global issue with various signs and symptoms that can have major consequences. It is important to note that bone quality such as fractures is not the only health risk to discuss with patients who have vitamin D deficiency. Other diseases include but are not limited to chronic pain (cancer, musculoskeletal, fibromyalgia); autoimmune, cardiovascular, and even neurologic systems are impacted.

The current thought is that vitamin D is more of a multifunctional hormone or prohormone. The early application of vitamin D as a key skeletal element has been augmented more recently by apparent extraskeletal effects of vitamin D. This is because vitamin D contributes to many processes in the body. Additional evidence suggesting that vitamin D is a hormone will be discussed in a section later in the article.

The purpose of this article is to provide information on the conversation if vitamin D is a vitamin and a hormone. It is also to provide information for frontline nurses, providing information on the different clinical manifestations, levels, and education for patient-centered care. Vitamin D is an over-the-counter drug that comes in

Austin Peay State University, School of Nursing, 601 College Street, Clarksville, TN 37044, USA
* Corresponding author.
E-mail address: ellisond@apsu.edu

Nurs Clin N Am 56 (2021) 47–57
https://doi.org/10.1016/j.cnur.2020.10.004
0029-6465/21/© 2020 Elsevier Inc. All rights reserved.

different types and different dosages. Some patients may be taking this without their physician's knowledge. Some patients may be taking vitamin D for hormone effects or vitamin effects. This aspect is important for frontline nurses in admission questions and documentation, medication reconciliation, and for education of patients in all settings.

OVERVIEW OF PATHOPHYSIOLOGY OF VITAMIN D

Vitamin D is a vital nutrient to maintain adequate health. It has the chemical structure similar to that of a steroid hormone and is actually similar to adrenal and sex hormones.[1] Vitamin D can be obtained from supplements and dietary intake, but there is also an endogenous form made in the body; however, all forms are not biologically active. The most common form, cholecalciferol, or vitamin D_3, is synthesized in the skin after exposure to ultraviolet B radiation or sunlight.[2–4] Ergocalciferol, or vitamin D_2, is the form found in plants, fortified foods, and some fish. Vitamin D must undergo 2 transformations, called hydroxylation, to become active for use in the body. The first conversion occurs in the liver, where vitamin D is converted to 25-hydroxyvitamin D [25(OH)D], also known as calcidiol.[2,4–6] Calcidiol is then primarily hydroxylated in the kidneys and converted to the biologically active form 1,23-dihydroxyvitamin D [1,25(OH)$_2$D] or calcitriol.[2,5,6] After the synthesis of vitamin D, it circulates by attaching to the vitamin D binding protein (VDBP). There are similar half-lives of both dietary and endogenous forms of vitamin D, ranging from 12 to 24 hours and depending on how quickly the liver converts it to 25(OH)D.[3]

VITAMIN D DEFINITION

A vitamin is any organic substance that is essential in minute quantities for nutrition in most animals and some plants. Vitamins act as coenzymes and precursors of coenzymes for regulating metabolic processes but do not provide energy or serve as building units. They are present in natural foodstuffs or are sometimes produced within the body.[7] As previously stated, vitamin D can be obtained from supplements and dietary intake, but there is also an endogenous form made in the body.

VITAMIN D HORMONE

A hormone is a chemical substance that helps control and regulate different activities in the body.[8] It is a "product of living cells that circulates in body fluids...and produces a specific often stimulatory effect on the activity of cells usually remote from its point of origin."[7] Many hormones affect certain target cells or organs in a different part of the body from than they are made or synthesized.[8] There have been many discussions on whether vitamin D should be labeled as a hormone rather than a vitamin. One source states that it is a prohormone, as the body converts the substance, vitamin D, into a hormone for it to be used.[9] Other sources state that Vitamin D is a hormone precursor, as it must be synthesized by the sunlight for activation.[10] Vitamin D is also the only vitamin that is, and can be, made by the body, unlike vitamins A, B, and C, that can only be found in food and supplements, providing further evidence that it can be viewed as a hormone rather than a vitamin.[6,11]

VITAMIN D: USES AS A HORMONE

Vitamin D plays a major role in neurobiological pathways and signaling cascades related to mental health as evidenced by the vitamin D response to certain elements and the vitamin D receptors (VDRs) in the brain. There is also evidence that vitamin D plays a part in the different endocrine pathways, reinforcing that a vitamin D deficiency can actually be a hormonal deficiency.[12] Furthermore, vitamin D has been found to be significant in brain development on a hormone level.[13] For this reason, there have been an increasing number of people using vitamin D as more of a hormone replacement rather than a vitamin supplement.

Several studies have shown that the use of vitamin D supplementation has a positive effect on autism spectrum disorder (ASD) symptoms, attention deficit hyperactivity disorder (ADHD),[14] and depression.[13,14] One study found that the frequency of depression was significantly higher in those with hypovitaminosis D because of the "decreased gross morphology, cellular proliferation, and growth factor signaling" and other hormonal abnormalities in the brain associated with the deficiency.[12] Another study discovered lower levels of vitamin D were associated with increased rates and severity of depression in the participants who did not receive supplementation of 40,000 IU of cholecalciferol once a week for 6 months. However, it is also noted that vitamin D seemed superior at preventing depression rather than improving the symptoms already acknowledged in the participants.[13]

VITAMIN D ASSOCIATION WITH DIFFERENT SYSTEMS OF THE BODY

Almost all cells and tissues in the body are now recognized as having VDRs, which is why it can be linked to other various systems and diseases.[5] Calcitriol, labeled as a hormone by many sources, is mainly known for its essential function of increasing the amount of calcium absorbed in the gastrointestinal tract and assistance in facilitating osteoid tissue mineralization.[11] In addition to helping the absorption of calcium in the intestinal tract, calcitriol also assists in the regulation of the parathyroid hormone (PTH) feedback loop associated with the calcium regulation that enables the mineralization of bone.[9] Calcitriol stimulates calcium reabsorption in the kidney's tubulars. In the skeletal system, calcitriol interacts with VDRs in osteoblasts and conjunctively with the PTH to control the turnover of bone. Not only is calcium and phosphorus absorption enhanced by calcitriol in the intestines, but PTH activity is also suppressed, inhibiting the proliferation of parathyroid cells and secretion of its hormones.[5]

Additionally, calcitriol has been shown to have enhancing effects on the immune system and other metabolic pathways. It assists in the production of cathelicidin and beta-defensin and modifies the production of certain anti-inflammatory cytokines; furthermore, there is evidence that it can increase activity in the lymphatic system and stimulate the production of insulin.[5,15] Because of high VDRs found in macrophages, T lymphocytes, B lymphocytes, and dendritic cells, many sources state that these findings support the theories that vitamin D has a role in combating different bacteria playing a fundamental role in preventing not only infections but also autoimmune diseases and chronic inflammatory states.[5,15] Calcitriol can also increase the phagocytic ability of the body's immune cells and reinforce the epithelial cells' functional physical barrier, especially in the corneal and intestinal barriers.[15] It is not surprising that a vitamin D deficiency has been linked to an increase in seasonal infections, such as influenza, given that it affects macrophage activation and production of antimicrobial peptides.[16] Because vitamin D helps cell maturity and can prevent rapid cell growth by activating certain genes, it has also been associated with the prevention of certain cancers, specifically breast and colon.[1]

The cardiovascular system and cardiovascular diseases have been heavily associated with vitamin D. There are either VDRs or calcitriol that are abundantly present in cardiomyocytes and the vascular and endothelial cells in the cardiovascular system.[17,18] Evidence has been found to link a deficiency in vitamin D to the progression of vascular calcification and atherothrombosis. This critical substance has been associated with the regulation of macrophage maturation and infiltration in the vascular system, resulting in the regulation of proinflammatory cytokines and adhesion molecules, which are crucial elements in atherosclerosis progression.[18] Increases in blood pressure related to an activity increase in the renin-angiotensin system have been directly related to vitamin D also.[19] Low vitamin D levels have been linked to resistant hypertension, or hypertension above target blood pressure despite strict adherence to 3 or more antihypertensive medications, because of the disturbances in metabolic actions such as glucose intolerance and insulin resistance and an increase in adiposity.[19] Furthermore, compared with those who had higher levels of vitamin D, individuals with a vitamin D deficiency were at an increased risk of developing a cerebrovascular accident (CVA) resulting from the known underlying cardiovascular risk factors that are associated with vitamin D such as diabetes mellitus and hypertension.[19]

Pain (also known as the fifth vital sign) is associated with vitamin D deficiency and can affect many body systems. Those can include but are not limited to musculoskeletal pain and cancer pain. Pain is one the body's most important, adaptive, and protective mechanisms for the body; therefore, it is important to understand the effects of vitamin D on pain.[20] Although the pathophysiology of pain and vitamin D remains unclear, observational studies suggest that vitamin D deficiency may contribute to the development of physical pain.[21] Physical pain is usually divided into nociceptive, inflammatory and neuropathic pain. Vitamin D levels have shown to have an impact on immune systems and anti-inflammatory effects that impact pain in many patients.[22] The anti-inflammatory effect in the body is by reducing the release of proinflammatory cytokines and suppressing T-cell responses.[22–24] Both observational and interventional studies have been researching the role of vitamin D in nociceptive and inflammatory pain. Nociception is the term used to describe how pain becomes a conscious experience and involves the normal functioning of physiologic systems.[20,25] Another example of vitamin D and pain is patients who suffer with fibromyalgia muscle pain. The presence of VDRs and vitamin D activating enzymes in the central nervous system (CNS) and effects of vitamin D on neurotransmitters have been suggested to explain the link between pain and vitamin D in patients with fibromyalgia.[26,27]

The immune system also has a connection with vitamin D. Vitamin D influences the adaptive and the innate parts of immunity.[22] For example, vitamin D is a potent inducer of antimicrobial peptides (AMPs) on mucosal surfaces and in immune cells.[22–24] AMPs constitute the first line of defense for invading bacteria and viruses on mucosal surfaces, including the respiratory tract.[22–24] In addition, vitamin D also affects T-cell responses and suppresses inflammation.[22] With vitamin D insufficiency, the immune system will move to a more inflammatory immune response involving Th1 and Th17 cells rather than Th2 and T regulatory cells (Treg).[24] Adequate levels of vitamin D, however, lead to less inflammation and lower levels of inflammatory cytokines and prostaglandins.[28]

There are numerous studies and research suggesting vitamin D is associated with the prevention and treatment of several chronic conditions such as type 1 and type 2 diabetes, multiple sclerosis, hypertension, and glucose intolerance.[6] Other evidence suggests that sufficient levels of vitamin D also have protective properties against the development of multiple sclerosis (MS) or lessens the frequency and severity of symptoms in those already diagnosed with MS.[29] Furthermore, vitamin D has been shown to help regulate adrenaline, norepinephrine, and dopamine, as well as serotonin depletion in the brain.[9]

CLINICAL IMPLICATIONS FOR NURSES

Because increasing numbers in the population have vitamin D deficiencies, it is imperative that more education is provided about the possible causes and what should be done to combat the declining levels of this pertinent substance. First, it is important to understand which vitamin D levels to obtain and monitor for adequacy. The most common level observed is calcidiol or 25(OH)D ,as there is a small amount that does not bind and remains free in the bloodstream. The half-life of this form is around 2 to 3 weeks, which also makes it a better indication if the vitamin D level is sufficient enough.[3,6]

Secondly, it is important to understand what the therapeutic level or range is of calcidiol. Although the recommended total circulating vitamin D level is not consistent among different agencies because of the variety of needs, such as race, age, geographic location, absorption, and synthesis issues, and other comorbidities, it has been found that most of the population can achieve adequate bone and overall health at levels greater than 30 ng/mL (75 nmol/L).[5,6,30,31] Suggestions for supplementation also vary based on the needs of the specific population but should be started if levels are shown to be below 20 ng/mL (50 nmol/L); for high-risk groups, supplementation is suggested if levels fall below 30 ng/mL.[5,30] It is further stated by the Endocrine Society and other studies that the optimal range of the 25(OH)D level is 40 to 60 ng/mL (100–150 nmol/L) to adequately maintain the functions associated with vitamin D.[5]

Lastly, the best sources of vitamin D must be understood. Little of the daily source of vitamin D comes from dietary intake, so it is important to understand good sources of dietary intake and how much UVB exposure and supplementation might be needed despite one's daily nutritional habits. Good dietary sources of vitamin D might be difficult to find for many, but some of the best sources can be found in **Box 1**.

Vitamin D synthesis by UV radiation can be affected by the season, time of day, length of exposure, amount of cloud cover, pollution or smog present, skin melanin, and sunscreen use.[6] On average, it is estimated that approximately 5 to 30 minutes of exposure 2 times a week is all most people need for vitamin D synthesis to occur. However, as stated before, because the varying environments and individuals, a consistent recommendation can be difficult to make.[11] Although a fair-skinned individual may only need a total of 15 to 45 minutes a week,[30] a dark-skinned individual, who have natural protection from the sun because of the higher amounts of pigment melanin in the epidermis, may need up to 3 to 5 times the amount of sun exposure to meet the necessary length of time for complete synthesis of vitamin D.[32]

Box 1
Good dietary sources of vitamin D

- Certain fatty fish (trout, salmon, tuna, mackerel)
- Cod liver oil
- Egg yolks
- Sardines
- Beef liver
- Fortified foods (milk, breakfast cereals, and orange juices)

Data from Refs.[5,6,30]

Table 1
Recommended daily vitamin D intake and tolerable upper limits

Age Group	Recommended Intake (Pludowski; NIH-b)	Tolerable Upper Limit (Pludowski)
Birth to 12 mo	400 IU	Up to 1000 IU/d
1–13 y of age	600 IU	Up to 2000 IU/d
14–18 y of age	600–1000 IU	Up to 4000 IU/d
19–69 y of age	800–1500 IU	Up to 4000 IU/d
>70 y of age	800–2000 IU	Up to 10,000 IU/d

Data from National Institutes of Health Office of Dietary Supplements (a). "Vitamin D: Fact Sheet for Consumers, 24 March 2020, https://ods.od.nih.gov/factsheets/VitaminD-Consumer/. Accessed 25 May 2020.

Recommendations on vitamin D supplementation vary mostly on age with comorbidities and necessity secondarily assisting in the amount that is recommended. The total vitamin D daily intake should be the combined total of dietary intake and supplementation. **Table 1** combines several agencies' daily recommendations for supplementation to include the maximum upper limit that should not be exceeded to decrease the chance of complications related to vitamin D toxicity.[5] It should be noted that overuse of supplements is almost always the cause of vitamin D toxicity and not excess sun exposure, as the body has the ability to limit the amount of the substance it produces.[9]

CLINICAL MANIFESTATIONS/EDUCATION...

As previously stated, vitamin D has many roles and functions in the body. There are many systems that a deficiency in vitamin D can also affect, including musculoskeletal, cardiovascular, endocrine, and neurologic. Although not as common, an overabundance of vitamin D can also cause various issues. Other than rickets, osteomalacia, and osteoporosis caused the decreased calcium regulation that vitamin

Table 2
Results of vitamin D abnormalities

Deficiency Serum Levels of 25(OH)D <20 ng/mL (50 nmol/L)	Toxicity Serum Levels of 25(OH)D >150 ng/mL (375 nmol/L)
• Rickets • Osteomalacia • Osteoporosis and osteoporotic-related fractures • Increase in cancers (colon, prostate, and breast) • Depression • Increase in infections, especially respiratory • Pain (musculoskeletal, cancer, fibromyalgia)	• Gastrointestinal (nausea, vomiting, weight loss, anorexia, constipation) • Endocrine (polyuria, polydipsia) • Neurologic (confusion, irritability, altered mental status, coma) • Heart arrhythmias • Hypercalcemia (depression, confusion, and leading to calcification of heart, blood vessels, and kidneys) • Hyperphosphatemia

Data from Refs.[1,5,26,30]

Table 3
Informational guide on vitamin D for the frontline nurse

Assessment Data	Health History-What to Look For!	Asking the Right Questions!
Subjective:	• Cardiovascular disease	• Do you take any over-the-counter vitamins?
• Health history	• Endocrine alterations	• If yes, were they prescribed by a physician?
• Functional health patterns	• Immune Disorders	• Why are you taking them?
○ Health perceptions	• Complaints of chronic pain	• What do they do for you?
○ Health management	• History of depression	• How much are you taking?
	• History of falls	• How often are you taking them?
	• Cancer	
	• Diet and exercise	
Assessment Data	Results of vitamin D toxicity with clinical signs and symptoms	Results of vitamin D deficiency with clinical signs and symptoms
Objective:	Serum levels of 25(OH)D	Serum levels of 25(OH)D
• Hypertension	>150 ng/mL (375 nmol/L)	<20 ng/mL (50 nmol/L)
• Laboratory Results	Heart arrhythmias	Rickets
• Medical Diagnosis	Gastrointestinal (nausea, vomiting, weight loss, anorexia, constipation)	Osteomalacia
• Objective signs and symptoms of pain	Endocrine (polyuria, polydipsia)	Osteoporosis and osteoporotic related fractures
• Diabetes	Neurologic (confusion, irritability, alter mental status, coma)	Increase in cancers (colon, prostate, and breast)
	Hypercalcemia (depression, confusion, and leading to calcification of heart, blood vessels, and kidneys)	Depression
	Hyperphosphatemia	Increase in infections, especially respiratory
		Pain (musculoskeletal, cancer, fibromyalgia)

(continued on next page)

Table 3
(continued)

Educating patients

Good dietary sources of vitamin D
- Certain fatty fish (trout, salmon, tuna, mackerel)
- Cod liver oil
- Egg yolks
- Sardines
- Beef liver
- Fortified foods (milk, breakfast cereals, and orange juices)

Recommended daily vitamin D intake and tolerable upper limits

Age Group	Recomended Intake	Tolerable Upper Limit
Birth– 12 mo	400 IU	Up to 1,000 IU/day
1–13 y of age	600 IU	Up to 2,000 IU/day
14–18 y of age	600–1,000 IU	Up to 4,000 IU/day
19– 69 y of age	800–1,500 IU	Up to 4,000 IU/day
>70 y of age	800–2,000 IU	Up to 10,000 IU/day

Educating patients

health management
goal to reach and maintain an adequate level of vitamin D in the body.
- Do not take more than the daily recommended dose of vitamin D without discussing it with your physician
- Report any change to your physician regarding dose taken
- Follow through with physician ordered laboratory tests
- Report any changes in your physical or mental condition to your physician
- Monitor diet - include or exclude sources of vitamin D foods as directed by a physician
- Manage the amount of sun exposure (10–14 min 3 x per week)

D assists, a vitamin D deficiency has also been linked to increases in infections, cardiovascular disease, and mental disorders such as depression.[9] **Table 2** provides an overview of signs, symptoms, and disease processes resulting from either a deficiency or overabundance of vitamin D.

SUMMARY

Vitamin D can be obtained for diet and direct sunlight. The most common form, cholecalciferol, or vitamin D_3, is synthesized in the skin after exposure to ultraviolet B radiation or sunlight.[2–4] Nevertheless, the thought is that vitamin D is more of a multifunctional hormone or prohormone. This is because vitamin D contributes to many processes in the body. Calcitriol has been shown to have enhancing effects on the immune system, the cardiovascular system, the endocrine system, and other metabolic pathways. There is evidence that vitamin D has also a role in depression, pain, and cancer. This is because all cells and tissues in the body are recognized as having VDRs.

The goal is to reach, and maintain an adequate level of vitamin D in the body. Frontline nurses care for patients who have single to multiple comorbidities. There is sufficient evidence that vitamin D impacts many systems in the body, and many people are prescribed or take over-the-counter vitamin supplements. There are an increasing number in the population who have vitamin D deficiencies; therefore it is imperative that more education is provided to nurses and patients. **Table 3** provides an information guide on vitamin D for the frontline nurse to summarize the critical information for knowledge and patient education.

CLINICS CARE POINTS

- Recommendations on vitamin D supplementation vary mostly on age with comorbidities and necessity secondarily in the amount that is recommended.
- The total vitamin D daily intake should include the combined total of dietary intake and supplementation.
- There are an increasing number in the population who have vitamin D deficiencies; therefore, it is imperative that more education is provided to nurses and patients.
- Those individuals taking vitamin D supplements should report and discuss with their physician dosage, amount, diet, and any changes in physical or mental conditions while taking the supplementation.
- Vitamin D is a vital nutrient to maintain adequate health, vitamin D deficiency is a global issue with various signs and symptoms that can have major consequences.

DISCLOSURE

Neither Dr. D.L. Ellison nor Mrs. H.R. Moran has any commercial or financial conflicts of interest or any funding sources.

REFERENCES

1. Siska G. Vitamin D is the new hormone. Pharmacy Times 2019. Available at: www.pharmacytimes.com/publications/otc/2019/OTCguide-2029/vitamin-d-is-the-new-hormone. Accessed May 24, 2020.
2. Raposo L, Martins S, Ferreira D, et al. Vitamin D, parathyroid hormone, and metabolic syndrome—the PORMETS study. BMC Endocr Disord 2017;17:71.

3. Muntingh GL. Vitamin D—the vitamin hormone. S Afr Fam Pract 2016;58(3):32–6.
4. Nguyen T. Vitamin D and vitamin D analogs. J Nurse Pract 2016;12(3):208–9.
5. Pludowski P, Holick MF, Grant WB, et al. Vitamin D supplementation guidelines. J Steroid Biochem Mol Biol 2018;175:125–35.
6. National institutes of health office of dietary supplements (b). "Vitamin D: fact sheet for health professionals24 March, 2020. Available at: https://ods.od.nih.gov/factsheets/VitaminD-HealthProfessional/. Accessed May 25, 2020.
7. Available at: https://www.merriam-webster.com/dictionary/vitamin. Accessed May 25, 2020.
8. Harding M, Kwong J, Roberts D, et al. Lewis's medical-surgical nursing: assessment and management of clinical problems. 11th edition. St. Louis (MO): Elsevier; 2020.
9. National institutes of health office of dietary supplements (a). Vitamin D: fact sheet for consumers, 24 March 2020. Available at: https://ods.od.nih.gov/factsheets/VitaminD-Consumer/. Accessed May 25, 2020.
10. Gittoes Neil. Vitamin D—what is normal according to latest research and how should we deal with it? Clin Med 2016;16(2):171–4.
11. Hinkle J, Cheever K. Brunner & Suddarth's textbook of medical-surgical nursing. 14th edition. Philadelphia (PA): Wolters Kluwer; 2018.
12. Föcker M, Antel J, Ring S, et al. Vitamin D and mental health in children and adolescents. Eur Child Adolesc Psychiatry 2017;26:1043–66.
13. Al-Batran, Talal M. Is there an association between Vitamin D and depression symptoms? Middle East Journal of Nursing 2016;10:22–5. https://doi.org/10.5742/MEJN.2016.92823.
14. Sotoudeh G, Rasi F, Amini M, et al. Vitamin D deficiency mediates the relationship between dietary patterns and depression: a case-control study. Ann Gen Psychiatry 2020;19(3). https://doi.org/10.1186/s12991-020-00288-1.
15. Sassi F, Tamone C, D'Amelia P. Vitamin D: nutrient, hormone, and immunomodulator. Nutrients 2018;10(11):1656.
16. Zmijewski M. Vitamin D and human health. Int J Mol Sci 2019;20(145). https://doi.org/10.3390/ijms20010145.
17. Wang T. Vitamin D and cardiovascular disease. Annu Rev Med 2016;67:261–72.
18. Nitsa A, Toutouza M, Machairas N, et al. Vitamin D in cardiovascular disease. In Vivo 2018;32:971–81.
19. Kheiri B, Abdalla A, Osman M, et al. Vitamin D deficiency and risk of cardiovascular diseases: a narrative review. Clin Hypertens 2018;24(9). https://doi.org/10.1186/s40885-018-0094-4.
20. Ellison DL. Physiology of pain. Crit Care Nurs Clin North Am 2017;29(Issue 4):397–406.
21. Wu Z, Malihi Z, Stewart AW, et al. Effect of Vitamin D supplementation on pain: a systematic review and meta-analysis. Pain Physician 2016;19:415–27.
22. Helde-Frankling M, Bjorkhem-Bergman L. Vitamin D in pain management, 2017. Int J Mol Sci 2017;18(10):2170. Available at: file:///C:/Users/ellisond/Downloads/Vitamin%20D%20in%20Pain%20Management.pdf.
23. Hewison M. Antibacterial effects of vitamin D. Nat Rev Endocrinol 2011;7:337–45.
24. Hewison M. Vitamin D and immune function: an overview. Proc Nutr Soc 2012;71:50–61.
25. Ignatavicius D, Workman ML. Chapter 3 assessment and care of patients with pain. Medical-surgical nursing: patient-centered collaborative care. 8th edition. St Louis, (MO): Elsever; 2016. p. 24–49. ISBN 978-1-4557-7255-1 VitalBook file.

26. Ellis SD, Kelly ST, Shurlock JH, et al. The role of vitamin D testing and replacement in fibromyalgia: a systematic literature review. BMC Rheumatol 2018;2:28. https://doi.org/10.1186/s41927-018-0035-6.
27. Makrani AH, Afshari M, Ghajar M, et al. Vitamin D and fibromyalgia: a meta-analysis. Korean J Pain 2017;30(4):250–7.
28. Gendelman O, Itzhaki D, Makarov S, et al. A randomized double-blind placebo controlled study adding high dose vitamin D to analgesic regimens in patients with musculoskeletal pain. Lupus 2015;24:483–9.
29. Rose A. What have we learned about vitamin D?" Medical Laboratory Observer 2017. Available at: www.mlo-online.com/continuing-education/article/13008897/what-have-we-learned-about-vitamin-d%20. Accessed May24, 2020.
30. Demer L, Hsu J, Tintut Y. Steroid hormone vitamin D: implications for cardiovascular disease. Circ Res 2018;122(11):1576–85.
31. Sakamoto R. Sunlight in vitamin D deficiency: clinical implications. J Nurse Pract 2019;15(4):282–5.
32. Nair R, Maseeh A. Vitamin D: the sunshine Vitamin. J Pharmacol Pharmacother 2012;3(2):118–26.

Enhancing Cognitive Function with Herbal Supplements

Shondell V. Hickson, DNP, MSN, APRN, ACNS-BC, FNP-BC *,
Linda K. Darnell, MSN, RN

KEYWORDS

- Prevagen • Gingko biloba • Acetylcholine neurotransmitter • Galanthus woronowii
- Cognitive function • Herbal supplements

KEY POINTS

- Dietary supplements, in general, are not FDA-approved. Under the law (Dietary Supplement Health and Education Act of 1994).
- Instruct patients that dietary supplements should be a part of their medication list.
- Herbs in their natural form are usually not as effective until synthesized with other properties.
- There are no dietary supplement that can reverse the effects of memory loss due to aging or other brain related diseases.

INTRODUCTION

Herbal medicine is the art and science of using herbs, for health promotion and preventing and treating illnesses that are not usually considered part of standard medical care. It is the leading therapy among complementary and alternative medicine (CAM) use in the United States.[1(p97)] An estimated 40% of adults and 11.8% of children have used some form of CAM therapy in the past 12 months.[2] Using herbal supplements to improve or stave off the effects of normal cognitive aging is appealing to many patients because of the misconception that "natural" therapies have no adverse effects. Herbal supplement manufacturers often saturate consumers with direct advertisement on various media platforms with alternative treatment of a variety of ailments, such as erectile dysfunction, diabetes, and weight loss, without mentioning its effects or proven efficacy. Take for example the commercial for Prevagen being advertised on radio.

School of Nursing, Austin Peay State University, P.O Box 4658, Clarksville, TN 37044, USA
* Corresponding author.
E-mail address: hicksons@apsu.edu

Nurs Clin N Am 56 (2021) 59–67
https://doi.org/10.1016/j.cnur.2020.10.005
0029-6465/21/© 2020 Elsevier Inc. All rights reserved.
nursing.theclinics.com

Radio Advertisement

"Do you have concerns about mild memory loss related to aging?
  Prevagen is the #1 Pharmacist Recommended Memory Support Brand. †
  You can find it in the vitamin aisle in stores everywhere.
  Prevagen. Healthier Brain. Better Life."[3]

It is not uncommon for patients to seek recommendations about herbal supplements from health care providers during their patient encounter. However, before responding, consider that most patients using herbal therapy or considering using them perceive them as efficacious and in some instances, more efficacious than conventional medicines.[4] Health care providers must assess the patient's cultural beliefs and obtain a comprehensive medical history due to the potential of adverse drug reactions before offering any advice or recommendations. The Dietary Supplement Health and Education Act of 1994 (DSHEA), requires for all dietary supplements (including herbs) carry on its label the statement: *"This product has not been evaluated by the Food and Drug Administration (FDA). This product is not intended to diagnose, treat, cure, or prevent any disease."* The purpose of this statement is to alert consumers that no evidence-based research or clinical trials were done to support the claims made by the manufacturers; therefore, caution is necessary.

PATHOPHYSIOLOGY OF NORMAL AGING COGNITIVE FUNCTION

Almost 40% of people older than 65 years, experience some form of memory loss. When there is no underlying medical condition causing the memory loss, it is known as "*age-associated memory impairment,*" that is, considered part of the normal aging process.[5] Cognition refers to all the process by which sensory input is transformed, reduced, elaborated, stored, and recovered. The domains involved with cognition include memory, language, perceptual motor, social cognition, executive function, and complex attention.[6(pp469–70)] Acetylcholine is the main neurotransmitter in the parasympathetic nervous system that is rapidly destroyed by a specific enzyme, known as cholinesterase. The degeneration of central cholinergic neurons impairs memory, and enhancement of cholinergic synapses improves cognitive processes.[7] Deficits in the neurotransmitter acetylcholine are thought to be responsible for memory problems.[8] Occasional memory lapses do not damage brain neurotransmitters, and symptoms can be corrected with simple interventions compared with degeneration of brain neurotransmitters and is irreversible and cannot be corrected. Degeneration of the neurotransmitters often leads to worsening brain decline, which results in diseases such as Alzheimer dementia or Parkinson.

Symptoms of Normal Aging Cognitive Decline

Normal age-related memory lapses are part of the aging process and do not disrupt work, hobbies, social activities, or relationships. Common symptoms include forgetfulness, difficulty remembering or learning a new task, losing things easily such as eyeglasses, or difficulty remembering someone's name or address. When these symptoms become disruptive, patients often seek help. Standardized evidence-based testing such as the mini mental examination can confirm or rule out neurocognitive disorders. If examination and testing is negative in neurodegenerative disorders, then patient education on management of symptoms should be integrated into the care plan.

EVIDENCE FOR HERBAL SUPPLEMENTS USE

It is inevitable that questions related to herbal therapy often occurs during the patient encounter process; therefore, health care providers must equip themselves with up-to-date knowledge on herbal therapy, particularly what is available and used to treat common illnesses. The most common herbal supplements used to enhance mild cognitive impairment include Galanthus woronowii, Prevagen, Ginkgo biloba, Panax notoginseng, Fructus lycii, and Polygala tenuifolia willd.[9] To determine the effectiveness of herbal supplements, several grading systems have been developed to provide clinicians with evidence-based methods to understand the mechanism, usage, and potential harmful effects of herbal therapy. The natural standard is a complementary medicine grading system founded by clinicians and researchers from more than 100 academic institutions.[10] It is designed to provide clinicians with the latest scientific data and expert opinions on complementary medicine including herbal therapies. It is a grading system to support the level of efficacy for a specific indication of the herbal supplement. The grading level ranges from A to F. A grade of A indicates strong scientific evidence, B is good scientific evidence, C is unclear, D is fair negative, and F is statistically significant negative evidence[1(p99)] (**Table 1**).

Galanthus Woronowii

Galanthus woronowii, also known as Voronov's snowdrop, is a class of Galanthus perennial plants from the family Amaryllidaceae.[11] This plant contains a natural alkaloid called Galantamine that has the ability to penetrate the blood-brain barrier and reduce the breakdown of acetylcholine and improve cognition in patients with Alzheimer disease.[12(p11)] Studies in animal model have concluded that galantamine improves cognitive functions by reducing amyloid plaque level in the brain, which causes memory problems.[13(p394)] Another animal study showed that early administration of galantamine reduces the preplaque phase in the brain, which causes the dementia symptoms. The drug galantamine suppresses oxidative stress, resulting in improvement of cognitive behavior in mouse model with Alzheimer disease.[14] The major side effects of galantamine are nausea, vomiting, diarrhea, dizziness, and agitation. This natural alkaloid forms the basis of the synthetic drug Galantamine, which is approved by the Food and Drug Administration (FDA) to treat mild to moderate Alzheimer disease. Whether this effect of this plant in its natural form results in increased clinical efficacy has not been demonstrated.

Prevagen

Prevagen is the number one selling memory supplement in drugstores across the United States.[15(p25)] Although Prevagen is not a herb, it is discussed because of its claim to improve cognition. The maker of this drug is Quincy Bioscience, and the active ingredient in Prevagen is apoaequorin, which is a protein isolated from the jellyfish *Aequorea Victoria*.[16] This drug is supposed to work by reducing increase calcium levels in the brain. High levels of calcium contributes to cell death, and the drug maintains healthy levels, thereby preventing dementia and improving memory.[16] The FDA, in a warning letter in 2012, alleged illegal marketing of the drug and that the active ingredient did not meet the definition of a dietary supplement. Prevagen's most commonly reported side effects were headache, dizziness, and nausea. Other less common events were memory problems, difficulty sleeping, and anxiety. There have also been a smaller number of reports of more serious potential side effects such as heart- and nervous system–related events. Prevagen cannot work to improve brain function because the active ingredient apoaequorin

Table 1
Herbal supplements for cognition enhancement

Herb	Therapeutic Use	Side Effects	Summary Findings
Galanthus Woronowii	Inhibits acetylcholinesterase thereby slowing the breakdown of the neurotransmitter acetylcholine	Nausea, vomiting, diarrhea, dizziness, and agitation	Galanthus in its raw has the potential to improve cognition by inhibiting cholinesterase
Prevagen	Decreasing calcium levels in the brain, which improves memory	Headache, dizziness, nausea, difficulty sleeping, and anxiety	Prevagen has no effect on memory because the active ingredient apoaequorin is destroyed on the GI track and has no effect on the brain
Ginkgo Biloba	Causes vasodilation and increases cerebral blood resulting in improved cognition and memory	Bleeding disorders Headache Impaired fertility Dizziness Diarrhea Constipation	Smaller and earlier studies have shown modest improvements in cognitive function Larger studies have not confirmed that Ginkgo biloba prevents memory loss or slows the progression cognitive decline
Panax Notoginseng	Reduces lipid deposition, oxidative stress, and inflammation in the brain that leads to cognitive decline	Dry mouth, flushed skin, rash, nervousness, sleep problems, headache, nausea, vomiting, and birth defects in animal studies	The active ingredient Panax notoginseng saponin has shown to have a role of antibrain aging
Fructus Lycii	Protects against neuronal injury and loss and enhances neurogenesis in the hippocampus and subventricular zone, improving memory and learning abilities	Hypoglycemia, hypotension, and in rare cases sensitivity to sunlight, liver damage, and allergic reactions	A study done on mice hippocampal neurons shows that Lycium Barbarum polysaccharides (LBPs) a major cell component has neuroprotective effect on cognitive and memory deficits by attenuating neuronal damage and inhibiting lactate dehyrongenase (LDH) release. Increased LDH activity and lactate are observed during aging and in Alzheimer's disease

| Polygala Tenuifolia Willd | Extract of polygala Tenuifolia (EPT) works by having some protective effects against neuronal death in the brain, thereby improving cognitive impairments | Hypoglycemia in patients taking diabetic drugs, overproduction of antibodies affecting patients taking immunosuppressant drug. Should be avoided in pregnant patients | Polygala tenuifolia can improve spatial organization and recognition, but it does not improve short- or long-term memory formation, as measured by free or cued recall. More research is needed to verify its effect on memory functions in aged animals |

is completely destroyed in the digestive system does not cross the blood-brain barrier.[17]

Ginkgo Biloba

Ginkgo biloba leaf extracts, also known as ginkogink, is an extract from the leaves of the ginkgo tree with the toxic ginkgolic acid removed. It is thought to stimulate prostaglandin synthesis, resulting in vasodilation, which increases tissue perfusion and cerebral blood flow, resulting in the therapeutic effect of improved cognitive ability, concentration, and memory. The National Center for Complementary and Integrative Health (NCCIH) lists the side effects of ginkgo biloba as headache, stomach upset, allergic skin reactions, and increased risk of bleeding in older and pregnant patients.[17] Ginkgo may interact with anticoagulants by increasing prothrombin time and can be poisonous if consumed raw or roasted.[18] Gingko biloba extract when taken at 80 mg twice daily with trazodone 20 ng twice daily may cause decrease in level of consciousness or coma state on the third day.[19(p2)] Ginkgo should be avoided in patients with epilepsy taking seizure medicines, such as phenytoin (Dilantin), carbamazepine (Tegretol), and phenobarbital. Several small, early studies showed modest improvements in cognitive function for older adults with dementia.[20] However, several larger studies have not confirmed that Ginkgo biloba extract prevents memory loss or slows the progression of cognitive decline or Alzheimer disease in older adults. In adults with normal cognition or mild cognitive impairment, Ginkgo biloba does not slow cognitive decline.[21]

Panax Notoginseng Saponins

Panax notoginseng saponins (PNS) are the main active compound extracted from the root of Panax notoginseng perennial plant. The active ingredient ameliorates learning and memory deficits in animals, probably by inhibiting oxidative stress and apoptosis and by stimulating neurogenesis.[22] A review of this plant demonstrates that it has antiinflammatory properties, antioxidation, and inhibition of neuronal apoptosis. It is speculated that PNS is a multitargeted agent with an antiinflammatory property in the adjuvant and alternative treatment of human chronic diseases. The analysis of the antiinflammatory and antiapoptotic effects leads to the preservation of brain nerves and regulates the activity and secretion of nerve cells, exerting antidepression and anxiolytic effects, which may provide new directions for further in-depth researches of related mechanisms.[23(p1)] The side effects of PNS includes dry mouth, flushed skin, rash, nervousness, sleep problems, headache, nausea, vomiting, and birth defects in animal studies. This is therefore not recommended for pregnant or breastfeeding patients.[22] In a study on mice evaluating the effects of PNS, it was concluded that there is potential to protect neurons from oxidative damage via attenuating the production of 8-oxo-2-deoxyguanosine, a biomarker of oxidative DNA damage, enhances the activities of antioxidant enzymes and the expression levels of uncoupling protein (UCP4) and UCP5 and protein that may be a promising agent in the treatment of dementia.[24(p6)]

Frutus Lycii

Frutus lycii also known as wolfberry/Goji is a ripe fruit of a deciduous shrub of the Solanaceae family found in Asia. The active ingredient in this plant is Lycium barbarum polysaccharide (LBP), which elicits neuroprotection to neurons stressed by A-beta peptides. An in vitro study showed that pretreatment of LBP to cultured neurons can effectively prevent A-beta peptide–induced apoptosis.[25] The side effects of Frutus Lycii includes hypoglycemia, hypotension, and in rare cases sensitivity to sunlight, liver damage, and allergic reactions.[26] An in vitro study was done on rats to determine whether LBP can elicit neuroprotection to neurons stressed by A-beta peptides. The results concluded that pretreatment of LBP to cultured neurons can effectively prevent A-beta peptide–induced apoptosis.[25] LBP has also been shown to improve memory and neurogenesis in rats, which in turn could be of benefit to patients suffering from Alzheimer disease and other forms of dementia.[27(p16)]

Polygala Tenuifolia Willd

Polygala Tenuifolia Willd, also known as Yuan Zhi or Senega root, is commonly used for a range of brain-related issues including stroke recovery anxiety, insomnia, depression, and degenerative conditions such as Alzheimer. Polygala tenuifolia supplementation may slightly increase cognitive ability in elderly people and has limited effect on cognition for healthy adults. Adverse effect of this drug includes hypoglycemia in patients taking diabetic drugs, overproduction of antibodies affecting patients taking immunosuppressant drug, and should be avoided in pregnant patients.[28] Supplementing Polygala tenuifolia can improve spatial organization and recognition, but it does not improve short- or long-term memory formation, as measured by free or cued recall. Much more research is needed to determine if Polygala tenuifolia qualifies as a nootropic.[29(p 6)]

SUMMARY

There is no known herbal supplement that can stop the effects of cognitive decline associated with normal aging. Although some herbs have shown promising results, it is not in its raw form. These herbs are broken down into tiny particles and specific isomers have been studied. Consumers should be warned that herbs should be used cautiously, and notifying health care providers is required in order to avoid drug interactions. Although an understanding of herbs is important, the preparation of herbs is key in considering its potency and effectiveness in treating a specific disorder. In certain preparations, the potency of the herb is strengthened and in others it is changed or nullified. Two major organizations that provide evidence-based information to assist consumers and health care providers are the FDA and the NCCIH.

The FDA is a federal organization responsible for protecting the public health by ensuring the safety, efficacy, and security of human and veterinary drugs, biological products, and medical devices and by ensuring the safety of our nation's food supply, cosmetics, and products that emit radiation.[30] Even though herbal supplements are regulated by the FDA, they do not fall under the category for drugs or foods but as dietary supplements. Under this category, dietary supplements manufacturers do not have to seek FDA approval before selling dietary supplements, and companies can claim that products address a nutrient deficiency, support health, or are linked to body functions if they have supporting research but they must include a disclaimer that the FDA has not evaluated the product.[30] If FDA finds that a dietary supplement manufacturer has significantly violated FDA regulations, FDA notifies the manufacturer in the form of a Warning Letter, and information about the supplement is also posted on the FDA Website for consumers.

The NCCIH has developed a fact sheet to assist consumers in their decision-making about complementary health products and practices. Its mission is to define, through rigorous scientific investigation, the usefulness and safety of complementary and integrative interventions and their roles in improving health and health care ("National institutes of health [NIH]," n.d.). Because the efficacy of herbal supplements may be questionable, further studies are needed by independent researchers to validate findings and claimed therapeutic uses.[4]

It is easy for consumers to become overwhelmed with the plethora of herbal supplements available when they enter almost any grocery or supplement store in communities throughout the United States. Herbal remedies are available without a prescription or any particular guidance except what the consumer may gather from the label, recommendations from friends, or other sources that may or may not be reliable. Therefore, it is important that nurse practitioners, nurses, and other health professionals are knowledgeable about herbal therapy and can discuss how they are to be used.

CLINICS CARE POINTS

- Lifestyle changes, a nutritious diet and exercise is the cornerstone approach to disease management.
- There are distinct differences between normal aging memory loss and dementia.
- Utilize evidence based assessment tools such as Memory Impairment Screen (MIS); Mini Mental State Examination (MMSE) tool, Montreal Cognitive assessment test (MoCA), diagnostic imaging and labs to rule out or confirm memory loss related diagnoses.

REFERENCES

1. Woo TM, Robinson MV. Pharmacotherapeutics for advanced practice nurse prescribers. 5th edition. F.A Davis; 2019.
2. Barnes PM, Bloom B, Nahin RL. Complementary and alternative medicine use among adults and children: United States, 2007. Natl Health Stat Report 2008. https://doi.org/10.1037/e623942009-001. PsycEXTRA Dataset.
3. Prevagen TV commercial, 'Concerns'. iSpot.tv. Available at: https://www.ispot.tv/ad/oDZ1/prevagen-concerns. Accessed June 8, 2020.
4. Zuckerman GB, Bielory L. The safety and efficacy of herbal remedies for atopic disorders remains uncertain. Int J Evid Based Healthc 2003;7(2):112–3.
5. Normal aging, mild cognitive impairment & dementia. Department of Neurology. Available at: https://www.med.unc.edu/neurology/divisions/memory-and-cognitive-disorders-1/faq/normal-aging-mild-cognitive-impairment-and-dementia/. Accessed June 8, 2020.
6. Norris DG, Kalm K. Chunking and redintegration in verbal short-term memory. J Exp Psychol Learn Mem Cogn 2019. https://doi.org/10.1037/xlm0000762.
7. Maurer SV, Williams CL. The cholinergic system modulates memory and hippocampal plasticity via its interactions with non-neuronal cells. Front Immunol 2017;8. https://doi.org/10.3389/fimmu.2017.01489.
8. Ferreira-Vieira TH, Guimaraes IM, Silva FR, et al. Alzheimer's disease: targeting the cholinergic system. Curr Neuropharmacol 2016;14(1). https://doi.org/10.2174/1570159X13666150716165726.
9. Eckert GP. Traditional used plants against cognitive decline and Alzheimer disease. Front Pharmacol 2010;1. https://doi.org/10.3389/fphar.2010.00138.
10. Natural standard. (n.d.). PubMed Central (PMC). Available at: https://www.ncbi.nlm.nih.gov/pmc/articles/PMC1250333/. Accessed July 6, 2020.
11. What you didn't know about snowdrops | Russian geographical society. (n.d.). Главные новости | Русское Географическое общество. Available at: https://www.rgo.ru/en/article/what-you-didnt-know-about-snowdrops. Accessed July 6, 2020.
12. Harland G. Snowdrop. London (United Kingdom): Reaktion Books; 2016.
13. Martins RN, Brennan CS. Neurodegeneration and Alzheimer's disease: the role of diabetes, genetics, hormones, and lifestyle. New Jersey: Wiley- Hoboken; 2019.

14. Saito T, Hisahara S, Iwahara N, et al. Early administration of galantamine from pre-plaque phase suppresses oxidative stress and improves cognitive behavior in APPswe/PS1dE9 mouse model of Alzheimer's disease. Free Radic Biol Med 2019;145:20–32.

15. Welch EL. Quackonomics! The cost of unscientific health care in the U.S. ...and other fraud found along the way. Conneaut Lake (PA): PAGE; 2020.

16. Apoaequorin & your brain | Cognitive vitality | Alzheimer's drug discovery Foundation. Alzheimer's Drug Discovery Foundation. Available at: https://www.alzdiscovery.org/cognitive-vitality/ratings/apoaequorin. Accessed June 8, 2020.

17. FTC & FDA issue warning letters to supplement sellers. Consumer information. Available at: https://www.consumer.ftc.gov/blog/2019/02/ftc-fda-issue-warning-letters-supplement-sellers. Accessed June 8, 2020.

18. Ginkgo. . NCCIH. Available at: https://www.nccih.nih.gov/health/ginkgo. Accessed July 22, 2020.

19. Góis R, Neto W, Silva C, et al. The use of the ginkgo Biloba plant and its interaction with other drugs. Proceedings of MOL2NET 2018, International Conference on Multidisciplinary Sciences, 4th edition. Paraiba (Brazil): Sciforum; 2018. https://doi.org/10.3390/mol2net-04-05542.

20. Victor S. Sierpina|Bernd Wollschlaeger|Mark Blumenthal. Gingko Biloba. AAFP American academy of family physicians. Available at: https://www.aafp.org/afp/2003/0901/p923.html. Accessed June 8, 2020.

21. Can ginkgo biloba prevent memory loss? . Mayo Clinic. Available at: https://www.mayoclinic.org/diseases-conditions/alzheimers-disease/expert-answers/ginkgo-biloba-memory-loss/faq-20058119. Accessed June 8, 2020.

22. Efficacy and safety of panax notoginseng saponin therapy for acute Intracerebral hemorrhage, meta-analysis, and mini review of potential mechanisms of action. (n.d.). PubMed Central (PMC). Available at: https://www.ncbi.nlm.nih.gov/pmc/articles/PMC4288044/. Accessed July 6, 2020.

23. Xie W, Meng X, Zhai Y, et al. Panax Notoginseng saponins: a review of its mechanisms of antidepressant or anxiolytic effects and network analysis on Phytochemistry and pharmacology. Molecules 2018;23(4):940.

24. Huang J, Jing X, Tian X, et al. (2017). Neuroprotective properties of panax notoginseng saponins via preventing oxidative stress injury in SAMP8 mice. Evid Based Complement Alternat Med 2017;1–7. https://doi.org/10.1155/2017/8713561.

25. Chinese herb list - information about traditional Chinese herbs. (n.d.). shen-nong.com - traditional Chinese medicine information, references & applications. Available at: https://www.shen-nong.com/eng/herbal/list.html. Accessed July 6, 2020.

26. Vitamins & supplements center. (n.d.). WebMD - Better information. Better health. Available at: https://www.webmd.com/vitamins. Accessed July 6, 2020.

27. Kwok SS, Bu Y, Lo AC, et al. (2019). A systematic review of potential therapeutic use of Lycium Barbarum polysaccharides in disease. Biomed Res Int 2019;1–18. https://doi.org/10.1155/2019/4615745.

28. Senega. Nova Pharmacy. Available at: https://www.novapharmacy.com.au/all-health-topics/herbs/senega. Accessed June 8, 2020.

29. Marlatt MW. Neurogenesis and Alzheimer's disease: biology and pathophysiology in mice and men. Curr Alzheimer Res 2010;999(999):1–9.

30. Fact sheet: FDA at a glance. U.S. Food and drug administration. Available at: https://www.fda.gov/about-fda/fda-basics/fact-sheet-fda-glance. Accessed June 8, 2020.

Herbal Supplements for Common Women's Health Issues

Angela Morehead, DNP, FNP-BC, RN*,
Leigh Ann McInnis, PhD, FNP-BC, RN

KEYWORDS

- Supplement • Alternative therapy • Women's health • Complementary therapy
- Menopause treatment • Premenstrual syndrome • Pregnancy

KEY POINTS

- Many women experience uncomfortable symptoms during menopause, and pharmacologic treatments have associated risks.
- Nausea and vomiting in pregnancy are common, and there are few Food and Drug Administration–approved pharmacologic choices for treatment.
- Premenstrual syndrome affects many women, and alternative therapies are promising for treatment.
- Many women stop breastfeeding because of insufficient milk supply, and some women use alternative therapies to increase their supply.

INTRODUCTION

The World Health Organization defines complementary or alternative medicine (CAM) as "a broad set of health care practices that are not part of that country's tradition or conventional medicine and are not fully integrated into the dominant healthcare system."[1] CAM is further defined by the National Center on Complementary and Integrative Health as "a group of diverse medical and health care systems, practices, and products that are not generally considered part of conventional medicine".[2] The use of alternative therapies, including supplements, has increased in the United States, with more than a third of adults reporting treatment with some form of CAM.[2] The use of CAM is especially prevalent in women, specifically in the reproductive years, with more than 67% admitting to any use of CAM in the last year. This figure includes more than 20% of pregnant women reporting CAM therapies.[2]

Nursing, Middle Tennessee State University, 1301 East Main Street, MTSU Box 81, Murfreesboro, TN 37132, USA
* Corresponding author.
E-mail address: Angela.Morehead@mtsu.edu

Nurs Clin N Am 56 (2021) 69–78
https://doi.org/10.1016/j.cnur.2020.10.006
0029-6465/21/© 2020 Elsevier Inc. All rights reserved.

nursing.theclinics.com

The National Center for Complementary and Integrative Health reported expenditures exceeding $30 billion per year on various forms of alternative therapies.[3] Most of these expenses are out of pocket, and the average spending on CAM increased as household income increased.[3]

Some forms of CAM are evidence based, but many are culture driven, and evidence to support them are often conflicting.[1] Women tend to obtain information regarding CAM from different sources that frequently do not include their health care providers. Providers must be aware of the most common CAM therapies for women's health, including their efficacy and adverse effects.[2]

MENOPAUSE

Menopause is the cessation of menstrual periods for 12 consecutive months.[4] Typically, the hypothalamus secretes gonadotropin-releasing hormone, which causes the anterior pituitary gland to secrete follicle-stimulating hormone (FSH) and luteinizing hormone. These hormones cause an ovum to mature, and during this time in the ovarian cycle, called the follicular phase, the follicles begin to secrete a fluid that contains large amounts of estrogen, which makes the ovum more sensitive to FSH. One ovum matures more rapidly than the others and starts to secrete larger amounts of estrogen, which suppresses the production of FSH. That mature ovum is then released to possibly be fertilized.[5] When a woman reaches menopause, the ovaries do not produce estrogen and do not respond to FSH, leading to cessation of ovulation and menstrual periods.[5] This process typically occurs naturally between the ages of 45 and 55, but can also be surgically induced by hysterectomy with oophorectomy, or removal of the uterus and ovaries.[4]

Common subjective complaints during this change include insomnia, vaginal dryness, dyspareunia (pain with intercourse), hot flashes, and night sweats.[4] There are also physiologic changes during this time, including vaginal wall atrophy, bone loss, and overall vasoconstriction.[6] Most of these alterations are due to loss of estrogen.[6] Women often complain of headaches, irritability, and depression during the time leading up to and including menopause. These symptoms affect as many as 50% to 75% of menopausal women.[7]

The management plan for menopause focuses on relief of symptoms. Women should first be counseled regarding lifestyle changes that could help with symptoms. These lifestyle changes include exercise, decreasing stress, and getting adequate sleep. Typical pharmacologic interventions include estrogen replacement, antidepressants, including selective serotonin reuptake inhibitors and serotonin-norepinephrine reuptake inhibitors, gabapentin, and clonidine.[6] Currently, the only medication approved by the Food and Drug Administration (FDA) for use to relieve menopause symptoms is paroxetine.[6]

Estrogen replacement helps to prevent bone loss and improves the lipoprotein profile, but these medications are not without risk. Estrogen replacement has been correlated with a small increased risk of breast cancer and thromboembolism, and it is recommended that it be used at the lowest dose and for the shortest duration as possible.[6]

When reviewing alternative therapies for menopause symptoms, it is important to note that the position endorsed by the North American Menopause Society states that hormone replacement therapy is the most effective. The position statement also maintains that although complementary therapies can be useful, the benefit appears to be similar to placebo.[7] Some of the most common alternative treatments for menopause symptoms are black cohosh and soy.

Black Cohosh

Black cohosh, or *Cimicifuga racemosa*, has been used by women who suffer from vasomotor symptoms (hot flashes, night sweats) during menopause. The mechanism of action is unknown, but it is thought to inhibit serotonin receptors.[8] Although it is the most widely used supplement to decrease vasomotor symptoms, there are mixed results from trials that have been done to determine efficacy.[7]

A study done to determine if the effects were dose dependent found that the patients receiving the highest dose had decreased hot flushes and sweating. In contrast, a study comparing an estrogen and progesterone combination to black cohosh found a decrease in symptoms in all groups. Still, the hormone group had a higher reduction in symptoms.[7] One randomized clinical trial found that compared with placebo, black cohosh did not reduce moderate to severe menopause symptoms.[9] Of note, a Cochrane review of black cohosh trials suggested that more research be done on the efficacy of black cohosh because of the significant variability of the available studies.[7]

Black cohosh is typically well tolerated, and the most common complaints are related to gastrointestinal upset. No carcinogenic effects have been found in animal studies, but participants in 1 human study exhibited elevated liver enzymes. However, this was a small study, and the elevation was later attributed to alcohol abuse.[7] Black cohosh is considered to be a safe, effective alternative therapy for menopause symptoms.[7]

Phytoestrogens

Phytoestrogens are compounds that occur naturally, often from food sources, and are plant based.[10] Phytoestrogens have effects similar to estrogen without the effect on the breasts or uterus and thus are considered by some a safer option for menopausal symptom relief.[7,10] When a woman has a low amount of circulating estrogen, such as during menopause, phytoestrogens have estrogenic effects. In contrast, when estrogen levels are high, they have antiestrogenic effects.[10]

There are 3 classes of phytoestrogens: isoflavones, lignans, and coumestans. The primary sources of lignans are flaxseed, vegetables, lentils, grains, and fruit.[11,12] Examples of lignans are enterolactone and enterodiol. There is conflicting evidence on the efficacy of lignans on menopausal symptoms.[11] However, some studies have shown beneficial effects on hot flashes with the use of flaxseed.[12] According to Cetisili and colleagues,[13] all participants using flaxseed had an increase in quality of life and a decrease in menopausal symptoms, although the greatest difference was seen in those that also received patient education about menopause.

In the isoflavone category, daidzein and genistein are 2 types of phytoestrogens. Soybeans, chickpeas, and lentils are some of the more powerful sources of these phytoestrogens.[11] However, there is conflicting evidence on the ability of isoflavones to produce a beneficial effect in menopausal women.[7,11] Daidzein requires a specific bacteria in the intestinal tract to an active format, and only 30% to 50% of women have this bacteria, with higher prevalence in Asians and vegetarians.[10] Although Hirose and colleagues[14] found that a low-dose isoflavone combination (genistein, daidzein, and glycitein) significantly alleviated symptoms of depression and insomnia in middle-aged women, It is important to note that Japan was the location of the study. Because it is known that this isoflavone requires the specific bacteria that is primarily found in the Asian population, it would be difficult to conclude that the effect found in this study is applicable to women who are not of Asian descent.

NAUSEA AND VOMITING IN PREGNANCY

Nausea and vomiting affect up to 80% of all pregnant women.[15] The cause of nausea during pregnancy is not known but is thought to be related to the extreme hormone changes that occur in the first trimester.[16] Typically, this condition subsides after the first trimester, but some women continue to have nausea throughout their pregnancy.[15] If this condition is severe and it persists, it can lead to dehydration, weight loss, and electrolyte imbalances. Severe nausea can lead to anxiety, depression, and overall lower quality of life.[16]

The typical nonpharmacologic recommendations for someone with nausea in pregnancy include small, frequent meals, reducing the amount of fatty foods or other foods that exacerbate symptoms, and eating when waking in the morning.[15] Patients should also be encouraged to stop smoking because this can increase nausea.[15]

Many medications are contraindicated in pregnancy because of the effects on the fetus, and complementary therapies are gaining acceptance. It is estimated that approximately 87% of pregnant women have used some form of alternative medicine during pregnancy.[16] The common therapies used include ginger and peppermint.[15] It is important to discuss possible side effects of herbal supplements with pregnant women because many alternative therapies have not been sufficiently studied to prove that they are safe for the fetus.[17] Most women assume that because the substance is natural that it is safe, and this is not always true.[17] Health care providers should consider the risks and benefits of alternative therapies before making a recommendation.

Ginger

Ginger has many medicinal applications, including alleviation of joint pain, treatment for osteoarthritis, and nausea and vomiting in pregnancy, chemotherapy patients, and postoperative patients.[16] The exact mechanism of action is still being investigated, but ginger increases gastric tone and motility and increases gastric emptying. In addition, it is known that chemotherapy drugs increase 5-hydroxytryptamine (5-HT), or serotonin, concentration. Serotonin is known to cause nausea by activating the vagus nerve. One of the actions of ginger was the inhibition of 5-HT effects, therefore decreasing nausea.[18]

Ginger can be used in many forms; it can be grated into food or tea, used as a syrup, or used in pill form.[15] When comparing ginger with placebo, multiple studies have demonstrated that patients had decreased nausea and decreased vomiting episodes.[15,16,18] Most studies that focus on ginger for nausea in pregnancy used varying amounts of ginger for the experimental group. The dose ranged from 500 mg to 1500 mg per day.[18] The difference in dose makes it difficult to determine if the effect is dose dependent, and what amount should be recommended to patients.

Ginger is considered a safe alternative therapy. However, a Cochrane review of patients who used ginger in pregnancy did note increased bleeding in the first and second trimester.[15,19,20] This increased bleeding has been attributed to a decrease in platelet aggregation resulting from ginger consumption.[18] For this reason, ginger is contraindicated close to labor or in patients who have a history of miscarriage.[19] It is important to note that there was no increase in spontaneous abortion or other birth anomalies noted in patients who used ginger for nausea in pregnancy.[19]

Peppermint

Mint is used as aromatherapy for its antispasmodic, lactation enhancement, and antiemetic properties.[21] It is also known to reduce fever, dysmenorrhea (painful menses), and diarrhea.[21] The mechanism of action is similar to ginger because it has antagonistic effects on serotonin receptors, and it is thought to act as a type of anesthetic on the stomach wall by inhibiting muscle contraction in the stomach.[16]

Peppermint is used in essential oil form, and the main components of the oil are menthol, menthone, and menthyl acetate.[21] Results from studies comparing peppermint to placebo for relief of nausea and vomiting are mixed. Most studies using peppermint aromatherapy have demonstrated decreased nausea and decreased vomiting episodes, but the difference from placebo has been insignificant.[16,21] It should be noted that 2 studies using controlled breathing revealed that although there was no difference between breathing in peppermint, isopropyl alcohol, or saline, that positive effects were felt by the groups using controlled breathing techniques.[21]

The FDA considers peppermint to be safe in pregnancy, and no adverse effects have been noted in any study.[21] Although it has not been demonstrated to be efficacious compared with placebo, it would not be harmful for pregnant women.

PREMENSTRUAL SYNDROME

Premenstrual syndrome (PMS) is a combination of physical and psychological signs and symptoms that occurs in the days preceding a menstrual period.[22] The cause of PMS is not known, but is likely due to the changes in estrogen and progesterone levels.[23] During the menstrual cycle, there are abrupt changes in these hormone levels; estrogen levels peak, then drop abruptly, then slowly increase. Progesterone levels increase and then drop.[5] During the luteal phase, approximately 7 days before menses, estrogen, progesterone, and serotonin levels decrease, and this affects some women with varying severity.[5] This theory has been supported by studies whereby women who were postmenopausal were given progesterone in cyclical doses and developed PMS symptoms similar to when they had been menstruating.[23] Studies have also reinforced that estrogen production is suppressed, and women have marked improvement in PMS symptoms.[23]

It is not known why some women are more affected than others, but symptoms of PMS are reported in approximately 30% to 80% of women.[22] These symptoms include bloating, mood swings, lethargy, irritability, breast tenderness, anxiety, sleep disturbance, and depression.[22]

Patients should first be encouraged to attempt lifestyle modifications that could help decrease PMS symptoms. These lifestyle modifications include regular exercise, reducing stress, and getting adequate sleep.[24] Current pharmacologic treatments for PMS include antidepressants, including selective serotonin reuptake inhibitors, serotonin-norepinephrine reuptake inhibitors, seroquel, and oral contraceptives.[22] It should be noted that these medications are not approved by the FDA for PMS treatment despite studies demonstrating efficacy.[23]

Damask Rose

Damask rose is known to have hypnotic, antiepileptic, and anxiolytic properties. It has been used to treat sexual dysfunction, depression, and stress.[22] It is grown primarily in the Middle East and can be made into an essential oil form for the treatment of the aforementioned conditions.[22] The mechanism of action is unknown, but the primary effect is on the central nervous system.[22]

Most studies investigating damask rose have not attempted to determine efficacy specifically for PMS, but instead for some of the individual symptoms of PMS, including sleep disorders, pain, depression, and anxiety. Heydari and colleagues[22] found that damask rose essential oil used during the luteal phase had a small positive effect on PMS symptoms. A questionnaire was used that covered the physical and psychological components of PMS. This study also noted that there were no adverse effects with damask rose, but did reference another study whereby nausea, vomiting, and headache were reported.[22]

Calcium, Vitamin D, and Magnesium

To understand the cause and thus treat PMS, vitamin levels during the menstrual cycle have been tracked. Decreased calcium levels, specifically during the luteal phase, and reduced vitamin D levels throughout the menstrual cycle have been reported.[25,26] As with other treatments, the exact mechanism of action is not entirely understood. Vitamin D has a role in the proliferation of some cells, but estradiol (one of the estrogens released during the menstrual cycle) releases enzymes that degrade vitamin D. The decrease in vitamin D is thought to contribute to PMS symptoms because a deficiency of vitamin D is associated with increased bloating and blood pressure changes. These changes are thought to be a result of the effect of vitamin D on the renin angiotensin aldosterone system.[25] Calcium deficiency during the luteal phase has been associated with depression, hallucinations, and restlessness.[25] Magnesium plays a central role in many body functions that can influence the response to the menstrual cycle, including blood glucose control, blood pressure regulation, and hormone receptor binding.[27]

One study done to determine PMS symptoms measured calcium, vitamin D, and magnesium levels during the luteal phase of the menstrual cycle and found that those participants with PMS symptoms had lower serum calcium and magnesium levels.[26] It should be noted that the serum calcium and magnesium levels were not below normal. However, they were lower than those participants in the control group without PMS symptoms.[26] Several studies have reinforced these findings; a 48% reduction in symptoms was reported from women taking 1200 mg of calcium once a day, and another study reported a greater than 60% improvement in symptoms with 1000 mg of calcium daily.[26] Of note, 1 randomized controlled trial found that PMS symptoms were reduced with calcium supplementation during the luteal phase, but not during the other phases of the menstrual cycle.[25] PMS symptoms can also be mitigated through increased dietary consumption of calcium and vitamin D.[25]

There are mixed results regarding magnesium levels and PMS symptoms. Khine and colleagues[28] found no difference in PMS symptoms between patients given magnesium supplements or placebo, but, as mentioned previously, Saeedian Kia[26] found that patients with lower levels of magnesium reported increased PMS symptoms. Similarly, another small, randomized controlled trial demonstrated reduced pain and mood changes with magnesium supplements.[27]

When compared with placebo, vitamin D, calcium, and magnesium are low cost and safe for use in alleviating PMS symptoms. The results in studies to determine efficacy are positive overall, and unless ingested in extreme amounts, supplements would not be harmful for a woman suffering from PMS.

LACTATION

Breastfeeding has long been established as the preferred method for infant nourishment. The current recommendation for breastfeeding is for at least the first 6 months of life.[28,29] Despite the known benefits, only about 37% of infants are breastfed exclusively for this timeframe. One of the most cited reasons for ceasing breastfeeding is inadequate milk supply. The most common pharmacologic agents for increasing breast milk supply are metoclopramide and domperidone.[29] These medications, also known as galactagogues, are not FDA approved, and no dosing information appropriate for lactation enhancement is available.[29]

Many breastfeeding mothers use alternative therapies to improve their milk supply. The most common herbal supplements for lactation include fenugreek and milk thistle. Of note, the American Academy of Breastfeeding (AAB) does not endorse any pharmacologic or herbal treatment for increasing the milk supply in a breastfeeding mother.[30] Despite the lack of evidence to support the use of these therapies, and the lack of support from the AAB, approximately 65% of lactation consultants report recommending n herbal treatment for increasing milk supply in lactating mothers.[30]

Fenugreek

Fenugreek is the most commonly used herbal supplement to increase breast milk supply.[29] Although the mechanism of action is not understood, 1 theory is that it stimulates sweat glands, and that the stimulation of the mammary glands (which are also sweat glands) in the breast is what leads to an increase in milk supply.[29,30]

There is minimal literature regarding the safety or efficacy of fenugreek, and the information is conflicting. One systematic review outlined the few trials that have been done and concluded that there is insufficient evidence to recommend the use of herbal galactagogues. Both studies that were referenced in the review quantified an increase in breast milk supply by either weighing the infant before and after feedings or measuring the milk produced by pumping. In addition, both studies compared the use of fenugreek to placebo.[30] One group of lactating mothers was given a fenugreek tea 3 times daily, and there was a significant increase in milk supply related to placebo. The other study compared fenugreek taken in capsule form to placebo, and no difference was noted between groups.[30]

No adverse effects were noted in the studies referenced above; however, fenugreek has been associated with nausea and vomiting and can contribute to diarrhea in infants.[30]

Milk Thistle

Milk thistle has been used in herbal mixtures for increasing milk supply. As with other herbal therapies, the mechanism of action is not known, but it is thought to increase secretion of prolactin, which increases milk supply.[31] The use of milk thistle to increase milk supply was supported by a study in which pregnant or lactating pigs were given milk thistle and a slight increase in prolactin was noted.[31]

There are limited studies regarding the efficacy of milk thistle for improvement in lactation. One study found that mothers who took a milk thistle mixture had a 50% higher milk production (measured by pumping) than those in the placebo group. The mothers in the treatment group also reported a longer duration of breastfeeding their infants.[31] Of note, milk thistle was just 1 component of mixture used for increasing milk supply; therefore, it is difficult to correlate milk thistle with the increase in milk supply.[31] Another randomized study comparing lactating mothers who took milk thistle supplements to placebo did not find a difference in milk production.[31] In 1 small study, the milk composition of mothers taking milk thistle while breastfeeding was determined to be the same as mothers taking a placebo.[32]

No adverse effects have been noted in breastfed infants whose mothers took milk thistle, and there is minimal excretion of milk thistle in breast milk.[31]

SUMMARY

Because many patients seek alternative treatments for various conditions, it is important for health care providers to be aware of the risks and benefits when recommending these as a therapy. A large number of patients perceive pharmacologic interventions as unsafe so they turn to complementary therapies. Patients often neglect to inform their provider about the use of supplements, and this could lead to dangerous interactions.

Although most alternative therapies are harmless, many have not been demonstrated to be efficacious when compared with placebo. More rigorous studies with larger cohorts are indicated to determine the safety and efficacy of complementary therapies. There are issues with many studies investigating alternative therapies, including high attrition rates, small cohorts, and having multiple confounding variables. The information on herbal supplements is primarily based on poor-quality research and anecdotal reports. Recommending supplements to patients should be done carefully because of lack of regulations in their manufacturing and lack of information regarding dosage.

DISCLOSURE

The authors have no disclosures.

REFERENCES

1. Barnes LAJ, Barclay L, McCaffery K, et al. Women's health literacy and the complex decision-making process to use complementary medicine products in pregnancy and lactation. Health Expect 2019;22(5):1013–27.
2. Johnson PJ, Kozhimannil KB, Jou J, et al. Complementary and alternative medicine use among women of reproductive age in the United States. Womens Health Issues 2016;26(1):40–7.
3. Available at: https://www.nccih.nih.gov/news/press-releases/americans-spent-302-billion-outofpocket-on-complementary-health-approaches. Accessed July 10, 2020.
4. Cash J, Glass CA. Family practice guidelines. 7th ediiton. New York: Springer; 2020.
5. Murray SS, McKinney ES. Foundations of maternal-newborn and women's health nursing. Maryland Heights (MO): Saunders Elsevier; 2019.
6. Peacock K, Ketvertis KM. Menopause. In: StatPearls. Treasure Island (FL): StatPearls Publishing; 2020. Available at: https://www.ncbi.nlm.nih.gov/books/NBK507826/.
7. Moore TR, Franks RB, Fox C. Review of efficacy of complementary and alternative medicine treatments for menopausal symptoms. J Midwifery Womens Health 2017;62(3):286–97.
8. Merchant S, Stebbing J. Black cohosh, hot flushes, and breast cancer. Lancet Oncol 2015;16(2):137–8.
9. Tanmahasamut P, Vichinsartvichai P, Rattanachaiyanont M, et al. Cinicifuga racemosa extract for relieving menopausal symptoms; a randomized controlled trial. Climacteric 2015;18(1):79–85.
10. Villa P, Amar ID, Bottoni C, et al. The impact of combined nutraceutical supplementation on quality of life and metabolic changes during the menopausal transition: a pilot randomized trial. Arch Gynecol Obstet 2017;296(4):791–801.
11. Santen RJ, Loprinzi CL, Casper RF. Menopausal hot flashes. UpToDate. Waltham, Mass: UpToDate. 2020. Available at: www.uptodate.com. Accessed July 13, 2020.

12. Sourinejad H, Dehkordi ZR, Beigi M, et al. The use of flaxseed in gynecology: a review article. Journal of Midwifery & Reproductive Health 2019;7(2):1691–711.

13. Cetisli NE, Saruhan A, Kircak B. The effects of flaxseed on menopausal symptoms and quality of life. Holist Nurs Pract 2015;29(3):151–7.

14. Hirose A, Terauchi M, Akiyoshi M, et al. Subjective insomnia is associated with low sleep efficiency and fatigue in middle-aged women. Climacteric 2016; 19(4):369–74. https://doi.org/10.1080/13697137.2016.1186160.

15. Argenbright C. Complementary approaches to pregnancy induced nausea and vomiting. Int J Childbirth Educ 2017;1(32):6–8.

16. Ozgoli G, Naz M. Effects of complementary medicine on nausea and vomiting in pregnancy: a systematic review. Int J Prev Med 2018;9:75.

17. Frawley J, Adams J, Steel A, et al. Women's use and self-prescription of herbal medicine during pregnancy: an examination of 1,835 pregnant women. Womens Health Issues 2015;25(4):396–402.

18. Lete I, Allue J. The effectiveness of ginger in the prevention of nausea and vomiting during pregnancy and chemotherapy. Integr Med Insights 2016;(11):11–7.

19. Lindblad AJ, Koppula S. Ginger for nausea and vomiting of pregnancy. Can Fam Physician 2016;62(2):145.

20. Shawahna R, Taha A. Which potential harms and benefits of using ginger in the management of nausea and vomiting of pregnancy should be addressed? A consensus study among pregnant women and gynecologists. BMC Complement Altern Med 2017;17:1–12.

21. Jouaeerad N, Ozgoli G, Hajimehdipoor H, et al. Effect of aromatherapy with peppermint oil on the severity of nausea and vomiting in pregnancy: a single-blind, randomized, placebo-controlled trial. J Reprod Infertility 2018;19(1):32–8.

22. Heydari N, Abootalebi M, Jamalimoghadam N, et al. Evaluation of aromatherapy with essential oils of *Rosa damascena* for the management of premenstrual syndrome. Int J Gynecol Obstet 2018;142:156–61.

23. Hofmeister S, Bodden S. Premenstrual syndrome and premenstrual dysphoric disorder. Am Fam Physician 2016;94(3):236–40.

24. Glickman-Simon R, Wallace J. Acupuncture for knee osteoarthritis, chasteberry for premenstrual syndrome, probiotics for irritable bowel syndrome, yoga for hypertension, and trigger point dry needling for planta fasciitis. Explore (NY) 2015; 11(2):157–61.

25. Abdi F, Ozgoli G, Rahnemaie FS. A systematic review of the role of vitamin D and calcium in premenstrual syndrome. Obstet Gynecol Sci 2019;63(2):213.

26. Saeedian KA, Amani R, Cheraghian B. The association between the risk of premenstrual syndrome and vitamin D, calcium, and magnesium status among university students: a case control study [published correction appears in Health Promot Perspect. 2016;6(1):54]. Health Promot Perspect 2015;5(3):225–30.

27. Schwalfenberg GK, Genuis SJ. The importance of magnesium in clinical healthcare. J Acad Chiropractic Orthopedists 2018;15(2):23–4.

28. Khine K, Rosenstein DL, Elin RJ, et al. Magnesium retention and mood effects after intravenous Mg infusion in premenstrual dysphoric disorder. Biol Psychiatry 2006;59:327–33.

29. Shawahna R, Qiblawi S, Ghanayem H. Which benefits and harms of using fenugreek as a galactogogue need to be discussed during clinical consultations? A Delphi study among breastfeeding women, gynecologists, pediatricians, family physicians, lactation consultants, and pharmacists. Evid based Complement Alternat Med 2018;2018:1–13.

30. Bazzano AN, Hofer R, Thibeau S, et al. A review of herbal and pharmaceutical galactagogues for breast-feeding. Ochsner J 2016;16(4):511–24.
31. Drugs and lactation database (LactMed). Bethesda (MD): National Library of Medicine (US); 2020. Milk ;Thistle. Available at: https://www.ncbi.nlm.nih.gov/books/NBK501771/.
32. Amer MR, Cipriano GC, Venci JV, et al. Safety of popular herbal supplements in lactating women. J Hum Lact 2015;31(3):348–53.

Herbal Medication to Enhance or Modulate Viral Infections

Sherin F. Tahmasbi, DNP, FNP-C[a],*, Maria A. Revell, PhD, MSN, RN, COI[a],
Natasha Tahmasebi, BSc[b]

KEYWORDS

- Viral • Herbs • COVID-19 • Immune • Gastrointestinal • Respiratory

KEY POINTS

- With the increase in globalization and ease of travel, being able to prevent and treat viruses has become a big issue in public health. Despite advances in treatment, viruses persist.
- Antimicrobial resistance places a significant burden on the US health system because several regimens with various classes of antibiotics may be required for treatment. This is a global health issue leading to researchers turning to plant-based interventions as a way to combat this problem.
- Herbal medications may provide some antiviral activities and defenses against increased viral load. This exploration also may result in more cost-effective interventions that have the potential to reduce mortality and economic losses.

INTRODUCTION

Viral infections and their emergence continue to impose a threat on human lives. Up to the present time, there have been limited numbers of vaccines that effectively work and few antivirals are licensed for use in clinical practice.[1] Added to this is the increase in antiviral resistance, meaning that drugs that do work are at risk of reduced efficacy.[2] The recent global pandemic of coronavirus 2019 (COVID-19) has provided evidence for the need of a preventative vaccination and effective treatment of viruses, with the United States having passed 9.4 million confirmed cases and a total death rate over 233,000 in November 2020. The aim of this article is to review some traditional treatments of viral infections, specifically addressing gastrointestinal and respiratory system viral infections, and in turn explore alternative herbal medications that are

[a] Tennessee State University, School of Nursing, 3500 John A. Merritt Boulevard, Campus Box 9590, Nashville, TN 37209, USA; [b] Kings College University, Guys Campus, Great maze pond, London SE1 1UL, England
* Corresponding author. PO Box 1712, Brentwood, TN 37024.
E-mail address: stahmasb@tnstate.edu

Nurs Clin N Am 56 (2021) 79–89
https://doi.org/10.1016/j.cnur.2020.10.007
0029-6465/21/© 2020 Elsevier Inc. All rights reserved.
nursing.theclinics.com

used in their treatment and the role that an advanced practice nurse plays in the administration of these medications. It concludes by addressing potential novel treatments on the horizon for these viral infections.

HERBS AND VIRAL DISEASES

Viruses play an important part in human diseases. With the increase in globalization and ease of travel, being able to prevent and treat viruses has become a big issue in public health. Despite advances in treatment, viruses persist. Vaccinations can take many years to develop after a viral outbreak. This is evident in influenza pandemics as well as the most recent COVID-19 pandemic.[3] As a result of viral evolution and the development of different strains of viruses, the efficiency of vaccines can be short lived.

Exploration of herbal medicines and the role that they play in treatment of viruses is necessary to potentially identify novel antiviral medications. Viruses differ significantly from bacterial infections (**Table 1**). Regarding bacterial infections, herbal treatments were the primary treatment options available before the use of antibiotics, many of which are derived from herbal plants. Overuse of antimicrobials used to treat bacterial, viral, and fungal infections, however, has led to the development of antimicrobial resistance and subsequent difficulty in treating these infections. Antimicrobial resistance places a significant burden on the US health system, because several regimens with various classes of antibiotics may be required for treatment. This is a global health issue, leading to researchers turning to plant-based interventions as a way to combat this problem.

OVERVIEW OF THE IMMUNE SYSTEM

The human body is attacked by millions of different microorganisms, such as bacteria, viruses, and fungi, every second. The human immune system is a complex organization that protects the body from these potential harmful organisms. The immune system performs this essential job in different ways, such as producing antibodies, killing infected cells, marking or killing microorganisms, and causing inflammation.

There are 2 types of immunity responses: innate immunity and adaptive immunity.[4] Innate immunity is inherited from parents and already is present at birth. Innate

Table 1
Differences between bacterial and viral infections

Types of Microorganisms	Virus	Bacteria
Survival	Requires host cell for survival	Living organism
Disease examples	Rhinovirus (the common cold), influenza, acute bronchitis, SARS, MERS, COVID-19, hepatitis A–E	Strep throat, pneumonia, urinary tract infections
Treatment	Vaccinations can help prevent viruses and antivirals can help slow the course of the infection in some cases	Antibiotics
Symptoms	Systemic, fever, and inflammation	Localized but can become systemic

Abbreviations: MERS, middle east respiratory syndrome; SARS, severe acute respiratory syndrome.

immunity is not antigen-specific, meaning it does not have any specialized defense systems for different types of pathogens.[4] Adaptive immunity develops in response to infections over the lifetime. Adaptive immunity is antigen-specific immunity.[4] Adaptive immunity reacts on the pathogens that it recognizes, and it is more potent than innate immunity (**Fig. 1**).[4]

The human self-defense mechanism contains 2 lines: the first line of defense includes physical, mechanical, and biochemical barriers; and the second line of defense includes the inflammatory response.[5] The first line of defense acts like a gateway, which prevents harmful organisms from entering the body. The 2 important parts of this gateway are the mucus membrane and skin.[5] The second line of the defense—inflammatory response—occurs as a response to tissue injury or infection.[5] The inflammatory response consists of many cellular and biochemical defense mechanisms. White blood cells (WBCs), however, play the most important role in the inflammatory response. The normal range of WBCs usually is between 5000 per mm^3 blood and 10,000 per mm^3 of blood.[5] The number of WBCs changes in response to different types of infection. WBCs are made in bone marrow and found in blood and the lymphatic system.

When pathogens pass the first barrier of the immune system—skin or mucus membrane—they enter the body, start using the body's resources, and rapidly increase their numbers. The immune system comes into action after the pathogens reach a certain number. Macrophages, mast cells, and innate lymphoid cells reside in the tissues at the site of the insult; these are the first types of WBCs, which intervene in the defense process.[4] Macrophages can cause inflammation by causing the blood vessels to release water into the infected area. Neutrophils are the next type of WBCs that enter the process of defense. Neutrophils also can kill healthy body cells in the defense process. The other type of WBCs that are involved in the defense process are dendritic cells (DCs). DCs act like the brain of the immune system; they save the data of pathogens in their memory and prepare different antigens.[6] DCs initiate adaptive immune responses.[6] Natural killer cells are the other type of WBCs, which are responsible for killing the body's defective cells, such as tumor cells or virally infected cells. Natural killer cells do not attack pathogens.[4]

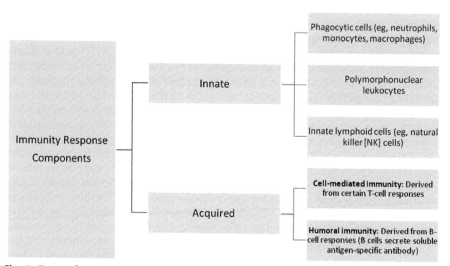

Fig. 1. Types of immunity responses.

The immune system is regulated by regulatory T cells, which secrete immunosuppressive cytokines to help control the immune response.[4] When antigen is eliminated or isolated from the body, the immune response resolves.

RESPIRATORY VIRAL INFECTIONS

Acute respiratory infections (ARIs) are the most common infectious diseases, primarily caused by viruses, and present clinically as upper respiratory tract infections and lower respiratory tract infections (LRIs). In 2014, LRIs were reported as the leading cause of deaths in the United States,[7] and influenza and respiratory syncytial virus (RSV) also are known to cause a high number of deaths.[8] When looking at the influenza virus, a majority of deaths across the world occur in people aged 65 years or older.[9] The United States was estimated to have had up to 62,000 deaths from influenza between October 2019 and April 2020.[10]

Current management for influenza consists of preventative vaccinations and treatment with antivirals. Both approaches have their limitations due to the virus' ability to mutate every year. These leaves the door open to the potential for pandemics of certain strains of the virus.[11] The neuraminidase inhibitors, zanamivir and oseltamivir, used in the treatment of influenza A, both have been found to reduce the duration of the symptoms in some cases but have not been found to be helpful when administered to healthy patients after 2 days of the start of symptoms.[12] There is an increasing amount of evidence to show that influenza viruses are becoming resistant to these neuroaminase inhibitors.[13] As a result of this and the significant possibility of many people losing their lives in the period between the virus mutation and development of a new vaccine for specific strains, which can take many months, the exploration of herbal medication as a means of management of influenza could be deemed reasonable. Many ancient civilizations used herbal medicines in order to both prevent and treat colds and influenza infections.[14]

In Japan, the use of the maoto has been administered traditionally to influenza patients. Maoto is a Kampo medicine, also known as a Japanese herbal medicine, composed of 4 medicinal herbs. A randomized controlled trial showed maoto granules given to patients with influenza had an equal efficacy to the neuraminidase inhibitors, zanamivir and oseltamivir.[15] Another herbal product that has been tested for use in individuals with influenza is echinacea. A randomized controlled trial conducted in the Czech Republic found that Echinacea was an early treatment given patients clinically diagnosed with influenza and was equally as effective as oseltamivir.[16] Traditional Chinese medicine (TCM) long has been studied for its therapeutic effect on influenza, and China continues to be a rich source for the production of novel antiviral medications. The TCM maxingshigan-yingiaosan (composed of 12 different herbal medicines) was studied in comparison to oseltamivir, as well as used in combination with oseltamivir, and both alone and together was found to reduce the time in which fever resolution occurred in comparison to patients receiving no treatment,[17] potentially suggesting that TCMs can be used as an alternative therapy in patients with mild forms of the disease. This study did not make clear whether the effects of the TCM were antipyretic or antiviral, however. Another benefit that was suggested promoted the use of TCMs, which were more economical than the use of Western medicine.[18] In order to consider the use of TCM in the practice of Western medicine, it is fundamental to understand their key ingredients and the effect that they have in order for their use to be evidence based as opposed to experienced based.[19] A recent animal study looking into Bai Shao, a Chinese herb, also known as Radix Paeoniae Alba, the white peony root, identified 3 compounds which it isolated from the herb. These 3 compounds were found to inhibit the activity of the influenza A virus in Madin-Darby canine kidney cells, leading to evidence for its use in clinical treatment of influenza.[20]

ARIs as a result of viruses are the primary cause of mortality and morbidity in children globally. One of the most major viruses causes ARIs in children is RSV. It is estimated that in the United States alone between 65,000 and 125,000 of children aged 2 years and under are hospitalized with the virus annually, with an estimated number of 65,000 deaths globally.[21] Ribavirin currently is the only approved antiviral used in the treatment of RSV. Currently, cost-effective and easily administered vaccinations and antivirals for the treatment of RSV are unavailable and, therefore, searching for a novel treatment of RSV is vital and herbal medicines provide a rich resource for this. A recent study researching the effects of the herbs, *Plantago asiatica* and *Clerodendrum trichotomum*, demonstrated that they had potential as antivirals in the treatment of RSV.

GASTROINTESTINAL VIRAL INFECTIONS

It is well known that hepatitis B can increase the risk of developing hepatocellular carcinoma, a leading cause of deaths due to cancer worldwide. Although hepatitis B currently is treated with antiviral drugs, its diagnosis often is associated with increased risk of hepatocellular carcinoma. Curcumin is an herbal medicine, derived from the plant turmeric, thought to possess anti-inflammatory and anticancerous activity without toxic side effects, with some studies showing that it may be useful in the prevention of hepatocellular carcinoma development from hepatitis B.[22] Many studies also have found that phytomal curcumin displayed promise in its ability to inhibit the growth of hepatocellular carcinomas through several different mechanisms, including the inhibition of vascular endothelial growth factor expression,[23] the protein associated with triggers the formation of blood vessels in cancer.

In Europe, it has been found that an estimated 52% of children use some form of complementary and alternative medicine (CAM), more specifically, herbal medicine.[24] The management of gastrointestinal disorders in both adults and children is particularly challenging and in more severe cases can lead to hospitalization. Many patients seek help from their practitioners; however, many treatments can be effective but lead to unwanted adverse effects and others may have fewer undesirable outcomes but may be less effective in treatment. A study looking into the reasons as to why parents give their children natural herbal medicine concluded that the primary reason was safety. Parents associated natural health products with being safe and, therefore, parents were more inclined to give them to their children as treatment.[25]

Every year in the United States, on average, norovirus is responsible for 109,000 hospitalizations and approximately 900 deaths (mainly in the ages 65 years and older population).[26] Due to the current lack of a vaccine for prevention of norovirus, preventative measures, such as good personal hygiene for food handlers, currently is recommended, but these have their limitations, such as increased expense of equipment and potential toxic effects from chemical exposure. Therefore, there is an increase in demand for more environmentally friendly chemicals. A study into the effect of 18 phytochemicals on norovirus found that curcumin and resveratrol were the top 2 most effective phytochemicals as antinoroviral agents.[27]

A recent review of herbal medicines and their effect on gastrointestinal disorders showed some positive results in their treatment, but the main limitation continues to be lack of clinical trials and, therefore, a lack of evidence-based information, preventing their use being recommended by medical practitioners and as a result, leading to the use of herbal medicines being primarily patient led.[28]

IDENTIFICATION OF VIRAL VERSUS BACTERIAL INFECTIONS

A major health issue in the United States and globally is antimicrobial resistance, in particular, antibiotic resistance. The primary cause of this antibiotic resistance is over-prescription by health care professionals and, therefore, overuse by patients, when in many cases the infection is not bacterial. It is estimated that antibiotics are prescribed unnecessarily in 30% to 50% of patients in hospital settings.[29]

Earlier detection and a more accurate diagnosis of these infections can allow for the prescription of antibiotics sooner for patients who need them as well as reducing over-prescription where unnecessary. It can be a challenge for health care professionals to distinguish between viral and bacterial infections because many of the symptoms present similarly. Currently, blood cultures, urine cultures, or spinal cultures as well as taking a thorough history can be used in order to diagnose a bacterial infection. The use of cultures enables profiling of pathogens from the blood; however, these tests sometimes can be limited because they are able to detect only a certain number and type of pathogens.[30] One study developed 7 genes as a means of discriminating between viral and bacterial infections, with 94% sensitivity and 59.8% specificity; further clinical authentication is required in order for this to be input into clinical practice.[30] Another recent study identified 11 genetic biomarkers in the blood that were successful in distinguishing between viral and bacterial infection 80% to 90% of the time. Although the main limitation of this study was the small sample size (94 adults), the findings still are significant and identify a potential means of reducing the unnecessary use of antibiotics which, should this move forward, would enable health care professionals to proceed in their treatment plan confidently in not using antibiotics.[31]

ROLE OF ADVANCED PRACTICE NURSE IN THE PRESCRIPTION OF HERBAL TREATMENTS

There still is debate as to whether nurse practitioners and other health care providers should be prescribing herbal medicine. One recent article discussed the points for and against the prescription of CAM, which herbal medicines can be classified as.[32] One argument for nurse practitioners learning about CAM as part of their training and being able to prescribe herbal medicines is that people who are choosing to use them often do so alongside the use of prescribed conventional medicine, often without telling their health care providers that they are doing so. This poses many problems, including the risk of potentially harmful interactions and contraindications. Therefore, it can be argued that it should be a mandatory part of a nurse practitioner's training to have an adequate level of understanding of potential side effects and uses of the herbal medicine or other CAM that patients may be taking, in order to design a safe treatment program with this in mind.[33]

Having said this, there also are many disadvantages to nurses being taught about CAM and prescribing herbal remedies to their patients. Primarily, there is extremely little evidence for CAM, meaning that even if they were to try and attempt to familiarize themselves with side effects and interactions, the lack of evidence would not permit this. As well, there are a huge number of concepts to CAM, making it difficult to make it part of a nurse practitioner's curriculum for training. Some investigators argue that it may be useful for nurse practitioners to refer to CAM practitioners, such as chiropractors or massage therapists, where they feel it would be beneficial.[32] In cases of herbal medicines, however, due to such a lack of evidence, many would agree that prescription of them without first knowing about their mechanism of actions, side effects, and contraindications absolutely should not be permitted and from the researched, discussed previously in this article, many successful findings often are in very early stages of research.

POTENTIAL TREATMENTS ON THE HORIZON

Despite development of various vaccines and therapeutic drugs, novel, mutant and resistant virus strains reduce their effectiveness. In an effort to increase possible interventions, alternative treatment options are important to explore. Herbal medications may provide some antiviral activities and defenses against increased viral load. This exploration also may result in more cost-effective interventions that have the potential to reduce mortality and economic losses.

A stage in the influenza cascade is the fusion of viruses with a host cellular endosomal membrane. This activity is promoted by low endosomal pH.[34] Vacuolar ATPase (V-ATPase) has been identified as a requirement for influenza replication.[35,36] This V-ATPase activity is responsible for pumping protons into endosomal compartments. Endomembrane organelle lumens, such as lysosomes, endosomes, secretory granules, and the Golgi apparatus, are acidified by V-ATPase. This acidification process is required for the influenza virus to enter the cell. It also has been reported that influenza viruses actually enhance V-ATPase function in order to promote infectivity.[37]

Maoto

Maoto is a traditional Japanese herbal medication that has been investigated for its effect on the influenza virus.[38] This herb traditionally is prescribed for upper respiratory infections or febrile diseases of an acute nature.[39] Maoto extract is developed from 4 plants: (1) ephedra herb (ratio 32.3% by weight), (2) apricot kernel (ratio 32.3% by weight), (3) cinnamon bark (ratio 25.8% by weight), and (4) *Glycyrrhiza* root (ratio 9.6% by weight).

It is hypothesized that maoto may have an effect on V-ATPase. The 2 components in maoto identified as having significant antiviral effects are cinnamon bark and ephedra herb. Their effects block the influenza uncoating process. This occurs through V-ATPase inhibition.[38] V-ATPases hydrolyze adenosine triphosphate to drive a proton pump. V-ATPases are key to various vital intracellular and intercellular processes, which include active metabolite transport, homeostasis, and neurotransmitter release.

Diphyllin

Diphyllin has been identified as a V-ATPase inhibitor. It can inhibit lysosomal acidification in osteoclasts.[40] Diphyllin is a natural compound isolated from the leaf extract of the *Cleistanthus collinus* plant. There has been an inhibitory effect of diphyllin against various viruses because research identified that it dose-dependently quenched acidic cytoplasmic vesicles within 20 minutes of incubation time. As a result of this finding, diphyllin could interfere with low pH–dependent membrane fusion that occurs between a specific virus and intracellular endosomes.

Diphyllin alters cellular-demonstrated susceptibility to the influenza virus and may have broad-spectrum antiviral activity, making it capable of addressing various viruses. This V-ATPase inhibitor has a safe therapeutic window. This suggests it as a potential broad-spectrum antiviral agent of high potency and lox toxicity.[41]

KIOM-C

KIOM-C is a total aqueous extract preparation that has shown promise in animal research. KIOM-C consists of the following: *Scutellariae Radix*, *Glycyrrhizae Radix*, *Paeoniae Radix Alba*, *Platycodon grandiflorum*, and *Ziniberofficinaletc*.[42] Research on mice demonstrated a reduction of viral titers and viral replication. KIOM-C induced antiviral states of significant strength to promote survival in mice against influenza A.[43] The KIOM-C formulation has been shown to have immune-enhancing and immune-regulatory effects.[44,45]

KIOM-C may be a feasible alternative antiviral therapeutic agent. It has demonstrated an ability to disrupt viral infection through type I interferon signaling molecules and proinflammatory cytokine activation. Based on in vivo results, treatment with KIOM-C can reduce influenza-induced mortality. This reduction occurred through its viral replication disruption and viral infection prevention by creation of an antiviral state in the lungs.[43] Additional research could expand identification of specific ingredients that induce antiviral effects as well as specific dose ranges for the best antiviral response. This ability to disrupt viral infection potentially could promote future use of KIOM-C in humans as an antiviral agent.[46]

Several viruses enter target cells based on pH. These include flaviviruses,[47] rhabdoviruses,[48] and coronaviruses.[49] Blocking V-ATPase activity by an intervention of herbal medicines may present an opportunity to impede influenza infections by preventing low pH–dependent membrane fusion. Virus replication also occurs and interfering with this replication could reduce viral load.

As viruses continue to evolve, vaccinations and other treatments based on predicted circulating strains are not as effective. These evolutions can render preexisting antibodies in the circulatory system from any earlier exposure ineffective. It is imperative to continue research to identify natural anti-influenza agents to expand the drug portfolio for clinical application. In addition to the use of herbal medicines in isolation, exploration of combination therapies in antiviral management also is important to investigate.

SUMMARY

The use of herbal medicines is particularly high in developing countries, meaning that a large percentage of the world's population relies on herbal medicine for at least primary health care. The research and evidence of some success in treating viral infections with herbal medicine, discussed previously, brings into question why it is not used more frequently as approved treatments in the developed world. One main reason is the lack of testing and little monitoring of patients' use of these medicines, meaning that their mechanisms of action and reason for sometimes effectively treating viruses, if at all, remains unknown.[33] Having said this, a recent study found that the prevalence of herbal medicine use in the United States is approximately 33%; with patients with more chronic conditions, such as stroke, cancer, and arthritis, found more likely to use them than those without.[50] This study also found that the main consumers of herbal medicine in the United States often use them alongside prescription and nonprescription medications. With this in mind, herbal ingredients appear to be a rich resource for the use of potential antivirals and the need to identify active ingredients, mechanisms of action, and potentially harmful side effects is necessary to move forward with incorporating their use into the health care system. Even if herbal medicines are not a cure, they may buy precious time in protecting and preserving life.

CLINICS CARE POINTS

The immune system becomes less effective with aging in different ways:
- Autoimmune disorders become more common as the immune system's ability in distinguishing self from non-self is reduced.[4]
- The number of lymphocytes that can respond to new antigens decreases—T cells respond more slowly to antigens.[4]
- Aging slows down the macrophages ability to destroy bacteria, cancer cells, and other pathogens. This can be a contributing factor to increased cancer incidence in older adults.[4]

DISCLOSURE

The authors have nothing to disclose.

REFERENCES

1. Howard CR, Fletcher NF. Emerging virus diseases: Can we ever expect the unexpected? Emerg Microbes Infect 2012;1. https://doi.org/10.1038/emi.2012.47.
2. Lin LT, Hsu WC, Lin CC. Antiviral natural products and herbal medicines. J Tradit Complement Med 2014;4(1):24–35.
3. Kelso JK, Halder N, Milne GJ. Vaccination strategies for future influenza pandemics: A severity-based cost effectiveness analysis. BMC Infect Dis 2013; 13(1):81.
4. Delves P. Overview of the immune system. Merck Manual Professional Version. 2020. Available at: https://www.merckmanuals.com/professional/immunology-allergic-disorders/biology-of-the-immune-system/overview-of-the-immune-system?query=innate. Accessed May,1 2020.
5. McCance K, Huether S, Felver L, et al. Study guide for pathophysiology, the biologic basis for disease in adults and children. Seventh Edition. St Louis: Mosby; 2015.
6. Dendritic cells. British Society of Immunology website. Available at: https://www.immunology.org/public-information/bitesized-immunology/cells/dendritic-cells. Accessed May 20, 2020.
7. El Bcheraoui C, Mokdad AH, Dwyer-Lindgren L, et al. Trends and patterns of differences in infectious disease mortality among US Counties, 1980-2014. JAMA 2018;319(12):1248–60.
8. Lambkin-Williams R, Noulin N, Mann A, et al. The human viral challenge model: Accelerating the evaluation of respiratory antivirals, vaccines and novel diagnostics. Respir Res 2018;19(1):1–15.
9. Thompson WW, Weintraub E, Dhankhar P, et al. Estimates of US influenza-associated deaths made using four different methods. Influenza Other Respir Viruses 2009;3(1):37–49.
10. 2019-2020 U.S. Flu Season: Preliminary Burden Estimates | CDC. Available at: https://www.cdc.gov/flu/about/burden/preliminary-in-season-estimates.htm. Accessed May 5, 2020.
11. De Vries RD, Altenburg AF, Rimmelzwaan GF. Universal influenza vaccines, science fiction or soon reality? Expert Rev Vaccines 2015;14(10):1299–301.
12. Cowling BJ, Chan KH, Fang VJ, et al. Comparative epidemiology of pandemic and seasonal influenza A in households. N Engl J Med 2010;362(23):2175–84.
13. Oh DY, Hurt AC. A review of the antiviral susceptibility of human and avian influenza viruses over the last decade. Scientifica (Cairo) 2014;2014. https://doi.org/10.1155/2014/430629.
14. Mousa HAL. Prevention and treatment of influenza, influenza-like illness, and common cold by herbal, complementary, and natural therapies. J Evid Based Complementary Altern Med 2017;22(1):166–74.
15. Nabeshima S, Kashiwagi K, Ajisaka K, et al. A randomized, controlled trial comparing traditional herbal medicine and neuraminidase inhibitors in the treatment of seasonal influenza. J Infect Chemother 2012;18(4):534–43.
16. Rauš K, Pleschka S, Klein P, et al. Effect of an echinacea-based hot drink versus oseltamivir in influenza treatment: a randomized, double-blind, double-dummy, multicenter, noninferiority clinical trial. Curr Ther Res Clin Exp 2015;77:66–72.

17. Wang C, Cao B, Liu QQ, et al. Oseltamivir compared with the Chinese traditional therapy maxingshigan-yinqiaosan in the treatment of H1N1 influenza: A randomized trial. Ann Intern Med 2011;155(4):217–26.
18. Xiaoyan L, Lundborg CS, Banghan D, et al. Clinical outcomes of influenza-like illness treated with Chinese herbal medicine: an observational study. J Tradit Chin Med 2018;38(1):107–16.
19. Han JN. Treatment of influenza: Chinese medicine vs. Western medicine. J Thorac Dis 2012;4(1):10–1.
20. Zhang T, Lo CY, Xiao M, et al. Anti-influenza virus phytochemicals from Radix Paeoniae Alba and characterization of their neuraminidase inhibitory activities. J.Ethnopharmacol. 2020;253:112671.
21. Respiratory Syncytial Virus (RSV) | NIH: National Institute of Allergy and Infectious Diseases. Available at: https://www.niaid.nih.gov/diseases-conditions/respiratory-syncytial-virus-rsv. Accessed May 8, 2020.
22. Teng CF, Yu CH, Chang HY, et al. Chemopreventive Effect of Phytosomal Curcumin on Hepatitis B virus-related hepatocellular carcinoma in a transgenic mouse model. Sci Rep 2019;9(1):1–13.
23. Pan Z, Zhuang J, Ji C, et al. Curcumin inhibits hepatocellular carcinoma growth by targeting VEGF expression. Oncol Lett 2018;15(4):4821–6.
24. Zuzak TJ, Boňková J, Careddu D, et al. Use of complementary and alternative medicine by children in Europe: Published data and expert perspectives. Complement Ther Med 2013;21(SUPPL.1). https://doi.org/10.1016/j.ctim.2012.01.001.
25. Pike A, Etchegary H, Godwin M, et al. Use of natural health products in children: Qualitative analysis of parents' experiences. Can Fam Physician 2013;59(8): e372.
26. Norovirus | Burden of Norovirus Illness in the U.S. | CDC. Available at: https://www.cdc.gov/norovirus/trends-outbreaks/burden-US.html. Accessed May 16, 2020.
27. Yang M, Lee G, Si J, et al. Curcumin shows antiviral properties against norovirus. Molecules 2016;21(10). https://doi.org/10.3390/molecules21101401.
28. Anheyer D, Frawley J, Koch AK, et al. Herbal medicines for gastrointestinal disorders in children and adolescents: A systematic review. Pediatrics 2017;139(6). https://doi.org/10.1542/peds.2017-0062.
29. Fridkin S, Baggs J, Fagan R, et al. Vital signs: Improving antibiotic use among hospitalized patients. Morb Mortal Wkly Rep 2014;63(9):194–200.
30. Sweeney TE, Wong HR, Khatri P. Robust classification of bacterial and viral infections via integrated host gene expression diagnostics. Sci Transl Med 2016; 8(346):346ra91.
31. Bhattacharya S, Rosenberg AF, Peterson DR, et al. Transcriptomic biomarkers to discriminate bacterial from nonbacterial infection in adults hospitalized with respiratory illness. Sci Rep 2017;7(1). https://doi.org/10.1038/s41598-017-06738-3.
32. Gardenier D. Should nurse practitioners prescribe complementary and alternative medicine? J Nurs Pract 2016;12(3):152–3.
33. Ekor M. The growing use of herbal medicines: Issues relating to adverse reactions and challenges in monitoring safety. Front Neurol 2014;4. https://doi.org/10.3389/fphar.2013.00177.
34. Stertz S, Shaw ML. Uncovering the global host cell requirements for influenza virus replication via RNAi screening. Microbes Infect 2011;13(5):516–25.
35. Müller KH, Kainov DE, el Bakkouri K, et al. The proton translocation domain of cellular vacuolar ATPase provides a target for the treatment of influenza A virus infections. Br J Pharmacol 2011;164(2):344–57.

36. Guinea R, Carrasco L. Requirement for vacuolar proton-ATPase activity during entry of influenza virus into cells. J Virol 1995;69(4):2306–12.
37. Kohio HP, Adamson AL. Glycolytic control of vacuolar-type ATPase activity: A mechanism to regulate influenza viral infection. Virology 2013;444(1–2):301–9.
38. Maoto. a traditional Japanese herbal medicine, inhibits uncoating of influenza virus. Available at: https://www.mdlinx.com/journal-summaries/influenza-virus-traditional-japanese-herbal-medicine/2017/08/30/7371625/. Accessed May 16, 2020.
39. Nishimura K, Plotnikoff GA, Watanabe K. Kampo Medicine as an Integrative Medicine in Japan. Vol 52. Available at: http://nccam.nih.gov/health/. Accessed May 16, 2020.
40. Sørensen MG, Henriksen K, Neutzsky-Wulff Av, et al. Diphyllin, a novel and naturally potent V-ATPase inhibitor, abrogates acidification of the osteoclastic resorption lacunae and bone resorption. J Bone Miner Res 2007;22(10):1640–8.
41. Chen HW, Cheng JX, Liu MT, et al. Inhibitory and combinatorial effect of diphyllin, a v-ATPase blocker, on influenza viruses. Antiviral Res 2013;99(3):371–82.
42. Chung TH. Effects of the novel herbal medicine, KIOM-C, on the growth performance and immune status of porcine circovirus associated disease (PCVAD) affected pigs. J Med Plant Res 2012;6(28):4456–66.
43. Talactac MR, Chowdhury MYE, Park ME, et al. Antiviral effects of novel herbal medicine KIOM-C, on diverse viruses. PLoS One 2015;10(5):e0125357.
44. Kim MC, Lee GH, Kim SJ, et al. Immune-enhancing effect of Danggwibohyeol-tang, an extract from Astragali Radix and Angelicae gigantis Radix, in vitro and in vivo. Immunopharmacol Immunotoxicol 2012;34(1):66–73.
45. Hu G, Xue JZ, Liu J, et al. Baicalin Induces IFN-α/β and IFN-γ expressions in cultured mouse pulmonary microvascular endothelial cells. J Integr Agric 2012; 11(4):646–54.
46. Kim EH, Pascua PNQ, Song MS, et al. Immunomodulaton and attenuation of lethal influenza A virus infection by oral administration with KIOM-C. Antiviral Res 2013;98(3):386–93.
47. Pierson TC, Diamond MS. Degrees of maturity: The complex structure and biology of flaviviruses. Curr Opin Virol 2012;2(2):168–75.
48. Albertini AAV, Baquero E, Ferlin A, et al. Molecular and cellular aspects of rhabdovirus entry. Viruses 2012;4(1):117–39.
49. Belouzard S, Millet JK, Licitra BN, et al. Mechanisms of coronavirus cell entry mediated by the viral spike protein. Viruses 2012;4(6):1011–33.
50. Rashrash M, Schommer JC, Brown LM. Prevalence and predictors of herbal medicine use among adults in the United States. J Patient Exp 2017;4(3): 108–13.

Herbal Medications Used to Treat Fever

Cheryl B. Hines, EdD, MSN, CRNA

KEYWORDS

- Herbs • Herbals • Fever • Pyrexia • Inflammation • Infection
- Traditional Chinese medicine

KEY POINTS

- Herbs can be used to blunt the release of inflammatory mediators.
- Herbs have useful antimicrobial properties and are finding new usefulness in light of escalating antibiotic-resistant microorganisms.
- Traditional Chinese medicine has used herbs for thousands of years to treat numerous febrile conditions by restoring the balance between the nonpathogenic and the pathogenic.

INTRODUCTION

Most of us have experienced fever at some point in our lives. Whether following exposure to a pathogen or triggered by immunologic responses, the symptoms of chills, shivering, sweating, thirst, aches, and fatigue are all familiar ones.[1] Normal body temperature is classically considered 37°C, but may vary 0.5°C to 1°C depending on individual and anatomic site from which measurement is taken.[2] Under normal conditions, the thermoregulatory center of the hypothalamus balances metabolic heat production and heat loss via respirations and evaporation.[2] Fever (pyrexia) is an increase in the hypothalamic set point, which is maintained by a series of pyrogenic and antipyretic pathways (**Fig. 1**). Heat is produced by neuronal activation resulting in peripheral vasoconstriction and shunting of blood to the body's vital organs and via muscle and hepatic metabolism. Fever is defined as a core body temperature of 38.3°C or higher.[2–4] Fever is a common symptom of numerous diseases and conditions (**Box 1**); therefore, this discussion limits its discussion of herbs for fever to 3 general areas: anti-inflammatories, antipathogenic, and those used in traditional Chinese medicine (TCM).

Capstone College of Nursing, The University of Alabama Tuscaloosa, 650 University Boulevard, Box 870358, Tuscaloosa, AL 35487, USA
E-mail address: cbhines@ua.edu

Nurs Clin N Am 56 (2021) 91–107
https://doi.org/10.1016/j.cnur.2020.10.008
0029-6465/21/© 2020 Elsevier Inc. All rights reserved.

nursing.theclinics.com

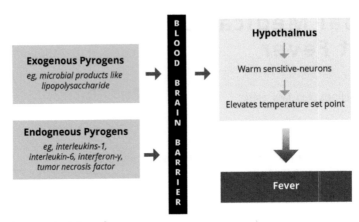

Fig. 1. Pathogenesis of fever.[3]

INFLAMMATION

After the physical barriers of our skin and mucous membranes, the inflammatory response is our body's next counter to tissue injury or infection. Rapidly initiated, inflammation is a complex generalized response involving the vasculature, plasma protein systems (complement, clotting, and kinin), and cellular mediators (**Fig. 2**). Fever is an inflammatory response that extends beyond the site of injury or infection.[3,4] Many herbals for treatment of fever work by blunting the inflammatory process (**Table 1**) or are considered herbal aspirins, as they contain some derivative of salicylic acid (eg, willow, meadowsweet, black haw, birch, black cohosh) and are therefore natural cyclooxygenase inhibitors.[14] In addition, anti-inflammatory herbs are rarely administered in an isolated manner. Rather, they are used in conjunction with other herbs or alternative therapies. **Box 2** provides some evidenced-based guidance for surface cooling, a technique many nurses use daily.

ANTIPATHOGENIC

Herbs have been used to treat infection for thousands of years. In northern Iraq, archaeologists discovered a fifty thousand-year-old skeleton buried with medicinal anti-infective plants.[15,16] Today, infectious disease remains a significant cause of morbidity and mortality worldwide. A classic symptom of infection is fever.[15] Infectious pathogens can be bacteria, fungi, protozoa, parasites, or viruses. Many herbs have bacteriostatic, bactericidal, or antiviral actions. In addition, they can work to boost

Box 1 Infectious and noninfectious causes of fever[3-5]	
Infectious	**Noninfectious**
Bacterial infections	Neurologic injury
Viral infections	Medications
Fungal infections	Immune-mediated processes
Parasite infections	Autoimmune disorders
	Postoperative stress
	Vascular thrombosis

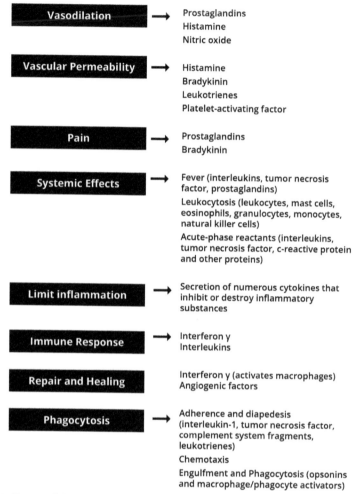

| Vasodilation | → | Prostaglandins
Histamine
Nitric oxide |

| Vascular Permeability | → | Histamine
Bradykinin
Leukotrienes
Platelet-activating factor |

| Pain | → | Prostaglandins
Bradykinin |

| Systemic Effects | → | Fever (interleukins, tumor necrosis factor, prostaglandins)
Leukocytosis (leukocytes, mast cells, eosinophils, granulocytes, monocytes, natural killer cells)
Acute-phase reactants (interleukins, tumor necrosis factor, c-reactive protein and other proteins) |

| Limit inflammation | → | Secretion of numerous cytokines that inhibit or destroy inflammatory substances |

| Immune Response | → | Interferon γ
Interleukins |

| Repair and Healing | | Interferon γ (activates macrophages)
Angiogenic factors |

| Phagocytosis | → | Adherence and diapedesis (interleukin-1, tumor necrosis factor, complement system fragments, leukotrienes)
Chemotaxis
Engulfment and Phagocytosis (opsonins and macrophage/phagocyte activators) |

Fig. 2. Mediators of the inflammatory process (cytokines). (Adapted with permission from Rote, 2019[3].)

people's immune or inflammatory responses.[6–9] **Table 2** is representative of several herbs that are used to combat fever that is associated with infection.

Attention should be given to the role of biofilm formation in the infectious process. The ever increasing and evolving problem of antibiotic-resistant microorganisms is of interest when considering the use of herbals alone or herbs in combination with antibiotics in the treatment of fever owing to infection.[26–28] Many microorganisms have specialized structures on their cell surfaces that assist with the creation of biofilms. Biofilms help bacteria to adhere to the hosts cells and tissues during the invasion stage of infection, thus allowing some bacteria to survive in what would otherwise be a hostile environment.[15,28] Biofilms are a structured colony of microorganisms that develop via the secretion of an extracellular matrix (polymeric substances), which provides strength and function to the colony. Biofilms are very difficult to eliminate and the source of many resistant or recurrent infections.[26,28]

Table 1
Herbs with anti-inflammatory activity

Plant Name	Actions	Plant Part Used	References
Chrysanthemum parthenium; Feverfew	Inhibits leukotriene production and the release of serotonin and histamine from platelets; inhibits NF-κB activity and cytokine secretion	Leaf	Goci et al,[6] 2013; Hartman and McEwen,[7] 2018
Curcuma longa; Curcumin, Tumeric	A natural COX-2 inhibitor; inhibits release of numerous cytokines	Root, rhizome	Goci et al,[6] 2013; Lee et al,[8] 2020
Echinacea purpurea; Echinacea	Reduces allergic and inflammatory pathways mediated by mast cells; suppresses cytokine production	Root	Gulledge et al,[9] 2018
Harpagophytum procumbens; Devil's claw	Inhibits both COX-2 and lipoxygenase pathways, resulting in the blunting of prostaglandins, cytokines, and serotonin	Root, tuber	Goci et al,[6] 2013; Menghini et al,[10] 2019
Liquidambar styraciflua; American sweetgum	Reduces oxidative stress and formation of free radicals; antiviral action	Leaf, seed ball, bark	Croson,[11] 2018
Salix alba; Willow bark	A natural salicylate (active ingredient in aspirin), nonselective COX inhibitor	Root	Desborough and Keeling,[12] 2017; Goci et al,[6] 2013
Zingiber officinale; Ginger	Inhibits macrophage and neutrophil activation; negatively affects monocyte and leukocyte migration; decreases proinflammatory cytokines and chemokine production	Root	Ezzat et al,[13] 2018; Goci et al,[6] 2013

Abbreviations: COX, cyclooxygenase; NF-κB, nuclear factor kappa-light-chain enhancer of activated B cells.

Box 2
Physical cooling in conjunction with antipyretics[5]

Do	Don't
Air-circulating cooling blanket style devices	Fans
Water or hydrogel circulating devices	Baths
Cool oral or intravenous fluids	Ice packs
	These strategies activate the thermal sensors in the skin, which antagonize the thermal set point in the hypothalamus. Heat-generating signals are sent, resulting in shivering. Shivering increases patient discomfort and oxygen consumption

Table 2
Herbs for fever associated with infection

Plant Name	Actions	Plant Part Used	Reference
Allium sativa; Garlic	Antibacterial (especially MDR bacteria); increases T lymphocytes and NK cells; virucidal; antifungal; antiparasitic	Bulb	Fritz,[17] 2019; Zhu and Zeng,[18] 2020
Aloe vera; Alovera	Inhibits viral replication (HSV-1); antimicrobial (gram-positive bacteria); stimulates macrophage and T-cell activity; promotes phagocytosis; stabilizes secreted cytokines	Leaf gel	Denaro et al,[19] 2020; Shedoeva et al,[20] 2019
Althaea officinalis; Marsh mallow, Hollyhock	Inhibits viral replication (influenza); antimicrobial; effective against MRSA		Denaro et al,[19] 2020; Mehreen et al,[21] 2016
Artemisia gmelinii; Wormwood	Antimicrobial (gram-positive bacteria); antifungal	Extract from aerial parts of plant	Mamatova et al,[22] 2019
Cinchona officinalis; Quinquina; Quinine bark, Peruvian bark, Jesuit's bark	Antimalarial (to a lesser extent with the increase of parasitic resistance), interferes with growth and reproduction of parasites	Bark	Noronha et al,[23] 2019
Eucalyptus sideroxylon; Mugga ironbark, red ironbark	Decreases viral replication; viral attachment inhibition; virucidal; anti-inflammatory actions	Leaf, bark	Ashour et al,[24] 2019; Denaro et al,[19] 2020
Syzygium aromaticum; Clove	Antibacterial; antifungal; antiviral; anti-inflammatory	Oils from flower buds	Gunawardana and Jayasuriya,[25] 2019

Abbreviations: HSV-1, herpes simplex type 1; MDR, multidrug-resistant bacteria; MRSA, methicillin-resistant *Staphylococcus aureus*; NK, natural killer cells.

Many herbs have antibiofilm activity, for example, *Herba patriniae* (patrinia, thlaspi, pennycress, white flower) is associated with inhibition of the gene expression responsible for biofilm formation, alterations in the microorganism's surface structure, and the prevention of mature biofilm development. These alterations greatly decrease the microorganism's ability penetrate the host's tissues and cause damage.[15,26] Tsukatani and colleagues[28] found that the ethanol extracts of several common herbs (eucalyptus, rosemary, and clove) were greater than 90% effective in eradicating the biofilm of numerous different bacteria. In addition, there were synergistic and/or additive effects when clove was used in combination with either rosemary or eucalyptus. Likewise, Hickl and colleagues[27] found that *Cistus creticus* ssp *creticus* (pink rock-rose, hoary rock-rose), *Rosmarinus officinalis* (rosemary), and *Salvia sclarea* (clary, clary sage) significantly inhibited biofilm formation of *Streptococcus mutans*, an anaerobic, gram-positive oral bacteria.

Free radicals also play an important part in the inflammatory process by facilitating the production of cytokines, and in the infectious processes, where they are produced during phagocytosis and pathogens destruction.[15,29] Thus, when treating fever caused by infection, herbs that are strong antioxidants have been proven effective in treating fever.

A free radical is an unstable molecule with an unpaired electron in its outer orbital. Free radicals travel throughout the body seeking out other electrons with which to pair. Because free radicals have low chemical specificity and are highly reactive, they can react with most any other molecule. Uncontrolled production of free radicals, for any reason but in this instance from the invasion of a pathogen, can lead to reactive oxygen species, oxidative stress, and tissue damage.[15,29,30]

Antioxidants, by contrast, are substances that can slow the cellular damage caused by free radicals. Antioxidants do this by donating one of their own electrons to the free radical (thus eliminating the problem of an unstable unpaired electron) without turning into a free radical itself. Our primary sources of antioxidants are dietary plants (eg, fruits, vegetables, and herbs).[29–31] Of particular antioxidant note are plants high in vitamins A, C, and E, and many polyphenols, such as phenolic acids, flavonoids, tannins, and lignans.[30,32] Although we are more familiar with fruits and vegetables that act as antioxidants, there are numerous herbs with antioxidant properties that are used to treat fever secondary to infection. Examples include *Artemisia afra Jacq* (African wormwood, wild wormwood), *Lonicera japonica* (honeysuckle), and *Andrographis paniculata* (green chiretta).[20,32]

TRADITIONAL CHINESE MEDICINE: COOLING HERBS AND HERBS THAT CLEAR HEAT

TCM has used the yin-yang theory of physiology and disease management for thousands of years. According to this theory, good health relies on the maintenance of balance between yin and yang. Therefore, regarding treatment of inflammatory and antimicrobial responses, the goal is to restore the imbalance between the nonpathogenic and the pathogenic, thus restoring the balance between yin and yang (herbs that clear heat).[33,34]

Within TCM, there are 4 qi (4 natures): cold, heat, warm, and cool, which reflect how healing herbs affect the proliferation or the impairment of yin or yang (**Fig. 3**). Thus, diseases with a heat pattern (fever producing) should be treated with herbs of a cold nature; likewise, diseases of a cold nature (create sensations of cold, eg, slow pulse) should be treated with heat-natured herbs.[34]

Furthermore, within TCM, herbals for fever are seen to clear interior heat and treat heat patterns. These medicinals are referred to as herbs that clear heat, and they work by draining fire, cooling the blood, resolving toxins, and/or by easing a deficiency of heat. Herbs that clear heat are commonly divided into 5 groups: (1) herbs that clear heat and drain fire, (2) herbs that clear heat and dry dampness, (3) herbs that clear heat and cool the blood, (4) herbs that clear heat and resolve toxins, and (5) herbs that clear deficiency-heat.[34,35] In no way is **Table 3** a complete collection of cooling herbs that clear heat; rather, it is a representative sample of herbs used to treat fever in TCM.

HERBS THAT CLEAR HEAT AND DRAIN FIRE

Heat implies the progressive nature of fire, with fire being the extreme of heat. Herbs within this classification are indicated for the treatment of febrile diseases caused by invading pathogens. Symptoms would include all those associated with infectious disease (eg, high fever, sweating, thirst, rapid pulse) as well as red tongue with yellow

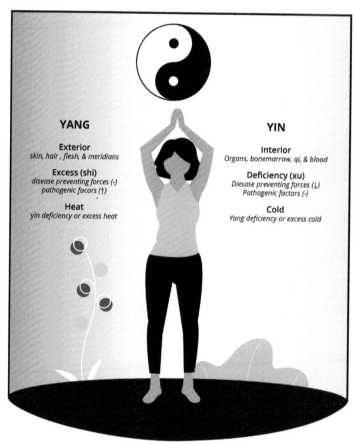

YANG

Exterior
skin, hair , flesh, & meridians

Excess (shi)
disease preventing forces (-)
pathogenic facors (↑)

Heat
yin deficiency or excess heat

YIN

Interior
Organs, bonemarrow, qi, & blood

Deficiency (xu)
Diesase preventing forces (↓)
Pathogenic factors (-)

Cold
Yang deficiency or excess cold

Fig. 3. Yin-yang theory in traditional Chinese medicine.[33,34] (Artwork by Kellie Hensley, graphic designer.)

coating.[34] An example of an herb to clear heat and drain fire would be *Herba comme-linae*, or the common dayflower. Sweet, bland, and cold *H commelinae* acts on the lungs, stomach, and small-intestine channels to resolve toxins, promote urination, and relieve swelling. It is indicated for initial treatment of the common cold, high fever, sore throat, swollen/sore carbuncles, edema with oliguria, and painful urination. It is can be boiled (15–30 g) with water for oral administration or applied topically as needed.[34,48]

HERBS THAT CLEAR HEAT AND DRY DAMPNESS

The treatment of damp-heat syndrome requires herbs that can clear heat but also address the unique symptoms of the body part affected. Damp-heat accumulating in the spleen or stomach may present as bloating, vomiting, diarrhea, and dysentery. In the colon, damp-heat may present as diarrhea, dysentery, or painful/swollen hemorrhoids. Accumulation of damp-heat in the liver or gallbladder may manifest as jaundice, reddish urine, or epigastric pain. Damp-heat is not limited to organs. Joint abscesses and skin conditions (eg, eczema and draining sores) are also conditions

Table 3
Heat-clearing Chinese herbs

Plant Name; Popular Name(s)	Actions and Indications	Cautions	References
Andrographis paniculata; Nemone chinensi, Andrographolide, Bhunimba, Carantina, Chiretta, Indian Echinacea, Justice, King of Bitters, Sadilata	Suppresses cytokines and inflammatory response Anti-inflammatory, antiallergic, immune-stimulating, antiviral. Suppresses influenza A Useful for acute respiratory infections, cough, sore throat	No serious AE, mild GI symptoms	Hu & Wu et al,[36] 2017; Muluye et al,[33] 2014
Coptis chinensis; Chinese goldthread	Inhibits tumor necrosis factor signaling, ↓ cytokine secretion and differentiation Antimicrobial activity against numerous bacteria, viruses, fungi, protozoans, helminths and chlamydia Useful for intestinal infections, gastroenteritis, cholera, dysentery, delirium due to high fever, skin diseases, conjunctivitis, otitis, hypertension, diabetes mellitus	Contraindicated in pregnancy, breastfeeding, infants, children as it contains berberine, which may slow hepatic clearance of bilirubin resulting in brain damage	Muluye et al,[33] 2014; Wua et al,[37] 2016
Herba taraxaci; Dandelion	Suppresses iNOS, COX-2, and production of pro-inflammatory cytokines Antimicrobial, antioxidant, anti-inflammatory, blood sugar and lipid regulation, hepatoprotective, diuretic effect Useful as an antipyretic, swelling, detoxification, and a variety of GI complaints (loss of appetite, dyspepsia, bile flow, GI upset)	Recognized as safe by the FDA as a dietary supplement. AEs are rare	Hu,[38] 2018

Flos lonicerae; Honeysuckle flower	Suppresses chemical mediator release (histamine, cytokines, granulocytes, macrophages, colony-stimulating factor, leukotrienes) Suppresses T-cell proliferation Bacteriostatic, bactericidal, antifungal, antimicrobial against oral pathogens Useful for infection, febrile diseases, antinociceptive, antidiabetic, antitumor, antioxidant, antiangiogenic, antipyretic, antiviral, hepatoprotective	Discontinue 7–10 d before surgery as has been found to inhibit platelet-activating factor	Guo et al,[39] 2015; Li et al,[40] 2015; Muluye et al,[33] 2014
Forsythia suspense; Forsythia	↓Anaphylactic antibodies, reduces mast cell degranulation, suppresses histamine release Antiviral, antimicrobial, antifungal, promotes bile secretion, antipyretic, hepatoprotective, antiemetic, diuretic, anticancer, and neuroprotective activities	No serious AE or toxicities reported	Huang et al,[41] 2019; Wang et al,[42] 2018
Houttuynia cordata; Fish mint, fish leaf, rainbow plant, chameleon plant, heart leaf, fish wort, bishop's weed	Immune-stimulating, anti-inflammatory, antibiotic, antiviral, diuretic, analgesic, hemostatic effects, antioxidative In rats, anticomplementary activity through classical and alternative pathways without interfering with coagulation Useful for pneumonia, bronchitis, colitis, urogenital infections, COPD, herpes simplex, SARS	No serious AE or toxicities reported Some allergic reactions have been reported with injectable forms	Lu et al,[43] 2018; Muluye et al,[33] 2014; Shingnaisui et al,[44] 2018

(continued on next page)

Table 3
(continued)

Plant Name; Popular Name(s)	Actions and Indications	Cautions	References
Isatidis folium; Isatis leaf	Anti-inflammatory effect due to strong inhibitory effect on COX-2 enzyme. Virucidal effect (in pigs) Bactericidal Useful for sore throat, redness of skin, antipyretic, encephalitis, acute dysentery, hepatitis, measles, pneumonia (bacterial and viral), influenza, epidemic cerebrospinal meningitis, encephalitis B, mumps, and diabetes	Chemically similar to aspirin	Liao et al,[45] 2018; Muluye et al,[33] 2014
Patrinia herba; Patrinia, Thiaspi, Pennycress, Whiteflower parinia, Dihurian patrinia	Prevents/inhibits the formation of biofilms. Decreases microbial exopolysaccharide production and swarming motility Antibiotic, hepatoprotective, sedating, hypnotic, mumps, antioxidant, antiviral, blood-activating and stasis-eliminating, promotes regeneration of liver cells, anxiety alleviating	None found	Fu et al,[26] 2017; Muluye et al,[33] 2014

Pulsatilla radix; Pasque flower	Anticytokine synthesis, inhibits proinflammatory cytokines Anti-inflammatory, antiparasitic, antimicrobial Useful for dyspepsia, premenstrual tension, psychosomatic disturbances, anaerobic non-spore-forming gram-positive bacillus, Crohn disease, selective growth inhibitor of intestinal bacteria	No serious AE or toxicities reported	Muluye et al,[33] 2014; Suh and An,[46] 2017
Radix isatidis; Banlangen, Isatis root, indago woad	Release inflammatory mediators from macrophages, such as NO, PGE$_2$, and proinflammatory cytokines Bacteriostatic Useful as an antibiotic, antidiabetic, immune-stimulating effects; encephalitis B and viral infections Influenza, SARS	Use with caution of allergic to aspirin	Liao et al,[45] 2018; Muluye et al,[33] 2014
Scutellaria baicalensis; Baikal skullcap or Chinese skullcap	↓ Mediators (cytokines) of inflammatory process: interleukins, histamine, tumor necrosis factor Antibacterial action against several common bacteria like *Helicobacter pylori* and *Escherichia coli*; some antiviral actions, but mechanism is unclear Useful as an antipyretic, antiallergic response, hepatoprotective, antihypertensive, diuretic, antibiotic, sedative (mild)	Hepatotoxicity and death (animal studies); contraindicated in pregnancy or breastfeeding due to ↓embryonic stem cell development	Muluye et al,[33] 2014; Webb,[14] 2006; Zhao et al,[35] 2019

(continued on next page)

Table 3
(continued)

Plant Name; Popular Name(s)	Actions and Indications	Cautions	References
Viola yedoensis; Japanese Arrowhead violet	Antimicrobial, inhibits viral replication of herpes simplex virus-1 and enterovirus. Cyclotides from Viola are effective in inhibiting HIV replication Strong inhibitory activity on inflammatory mediators (NO, cytokines and iNOS) Antibiotic, anti-inflammatory, antipyretic, skin disease (eczema, impetigo, acne, pruritus, cradle cap); URIs with fever	No serious AE or toxicities reported	Jeong et al,[47] 2016; Muluye et al,[33] 2014

Abbreviations: AE, adverse effects; COPD, chronic obstructive pulmonary disease; COX-2, cyclooxygenase 2; FDA Food and Drug Administration; GI, gastrointestinal; HIV, human immunodeficiency virus; iNOS, inducible nitric oxide synthase; NO, nitric oxide; PGE_2, prostaglandin E2; SARS, severe acute respiratory syndrome; URI, upper respiratory infections.

of damp-heat. Because these medications are considered to have bitter-cold proper-ties, high (toxic) doses can damage the stomach and consume yin. Therefore, doses should be small and stomach assessments frequent.[34] An example of an herb to clear heat and dry dampness is *Cortex fraxini* (ash bark). This slightly acidic-bitter, cold herb acts on the liver, gallbladder, and large-intestine channels. It is indicated for damp-heat diarrhea or dysentery, red or white vaginal discharge and or itching, and red eye with swelling and pain.[34,49]

HERBS THAT CLEAR HEAT AND RESOLVE TOXINS

As the name implies, the herbals within this classification are indicated for the treat-ment of bacterial infections, but also mumps, sore throat, diarrhea due to toxins, in-sect or snake bite, cancer, burns, and other acute febrile diseases. Care should be taken to choose the herb or combination of herbs best suited to the clinical manifes-tations. Because these herbs can damage the spleen and stomach, their use should be discontinued as soon as therapeutic effect is achieved. *Flos chrysanthemi indici* (wild chrysanthemum flower) is an herb that clears heat and resolves toxins. The dried flower head is boiled (9–15 g) as an oral dose or made into an ointment for dermal application. It is a bitter, strong-tasting herb with a slight cold action. It works on the liver and heart channels, clearing heat, resolving toxins, draining fire, and calming the liver. It is indicated for deep skin boils, sores, or carbuncles with swelling. It is also used to relieve throat pain caused by the buildup of heat toxins. It should be used cautiously in pregnancy.[34,50,51]

HERBS THAT CLEAR HEAT AND COOL THE BLOOD

Working from the premise that the heart controls the blood and the liver stores the blood, herbs that clear heat and cool the blood primarily work on the heart and liver. Cold and either bitter or salty in nature, these herbs help clear and resolve pathogenic heat in warm febrile diseases, heat caused by nutritional imbalances, and disharmony in the heart spirit. Symptoms may include crimson tongue, fever aggravated at night, difficulty sleeping, rapid and weak pulse, delirium, and even coma. Barely visible macules and papules may occur as well as evidence of blood from body orifices and fluids. An example of an herb that clears heat and cools the blood is *Radix paeoniae rubra*, or red peony root. This bitter, slightly cold herb acts on liver channels to clear heat, cool the blood, allay blood stasis, and relieve pain. *R paeoniae rubra* is used to treat macules and papules related to nutritional imbal-ance, blood-spitting and nosebleed, swollen sores and ulcers, liver-depressed hypochondriac pain, premenstrual symptoms, menstrual pain, and abdominal pain and injury from trauma.[34,52,53]

HERBS THAT CLEAR HEAT FROM DEFICIENCY

The primary role of herbs that clear heat from deficiency is to treat deficiency-heat syndrome with steaming bone fever, a deep internal heat arising from severe yin defi-ciency. Conditions treated with this class of herbs are fevers of the afternoon, night, night sweats, sleeplessness, and excess-heat syndrome. *Herba artemisiae annuae*, sweet wormwood, is bitter and pungent. In autumn, old stems are removed and dried in the shade. The stems are boiled (6–12 g) in water, or juice can be extracted from fresh stems. Both preparations are taken orally to treat steaming bone fever, resolve summer heat, prevent malaria attacks, and relieve jaundice.[14,34,54]

SUMMARY

Fever is a complex physiologic response, and yet it is commonplace and afflicts people across the lifespan. Herbs and plant-based medicines have been used throughout history to treat fever. Deciding which herbal remedies to use often depends on the cause of the fever, what is available geographically, and traditions within the individual's culture.

CLINICS CARE POINTS

- Fever is a normal body defense mechanism.[2,5]
- Fever can be infectious or non-infectious in origin.[2,5]
- Incorporation of non-pharmacologic therapies, non-herbal therapies are also important to wellness.[5]
- Often treatment of fever is focused on restoring the body to homeostasis.[33]
- Poly-herbal therapy can have synergistic effects with herbal and non-herbal treatments.[5,20,33]

DISCLOSURE

The author has nothing to disclose.

REFERENCES

1. Ames NJ, Powers JH, Ranucci A, et al. A systematic approach for studying the signs and symptoms of fever in adult patients: the fever assessment tool (FAST). Health Qual Life Outcomes 2017;15(1):1–11. Available at: https://doaj.org/article/f3c022210b184a5d91341d19f00676e8.
2. Steele GM, Franco-Paredes C, Chastain DB. Noninfectious causes of fever in adults. Nurse Pract 2018;43(4):38–44.
3. Rote NS. Innate immunity: inflammation and wound healing. In: McCance KL, Huether SE, editors. Pathophysiology: the biologic basis for disease in adults and children. 8th edition. St. Louis (MO): Elsevier; 2019. p. 191–209.
4. Ladha E, House-Kokan M, Gillespie M. The ABCCs of sepsis: a framework for understanding the pathophysiology of sepsis. Can J Crit Care Nurs 2019;30(4): 12–21.
5. Schell-Chaple H. Fever suppression in patients with infection: state of the evidence. Nursing 2018 Critical Care 2018;13(5):6–13.
6. Goci E, Shkreli R, Haloci E, et al. Complementary and alternative medicine (CAM) for pain, herbal anti-inflammatory drugs. Eur Sci J 2013;9(9):90–105.
7. Hartmann G, McEwen B. The potential of herbal medicine in the management of endometriosis. Journal of the Australian Traditional-Medicine Society 2018;24(3): 146–54.
8. Lee S-Y, Cho S-S, Li YC, et al. Anti-inflammatory effect of Curcuma longa and Allium hookeri co-treatment via NR-κB and COX-2 pathways. Sci Rep 2020;10: 1–11. Available at: https://www.nature.com/articles/s41598-020-62749-7.
9. Gulledge TV, Collette NM, Mackey E, et al. Mast cell degranulation and calcium influx are inhibited by Echinacea purpurea extract and the alkylamide dodeca-2E,4E-dienoic acid isobutylamide. J Ethnopharmacol 2018;212:166–74.
10. Menghini L, Recinella L, Leone S, et al. Devil's claw (Harpagophytum procumbens) and chronic inflammatory diseases: a concise overview on preclinical and clinical data. Phytother Res 2019;33:2152–62.

11. Croson L. Forest gold: anti-inflammatory properties of Liquidambar styraciflua (American sweetgum). Journal of the American Herbalists Guild 2018;16(1): 78–87.

12. Desborough MJR, Keeling DM. The aspirin story-from willow to wonder drug. Br J Haematol 2017;177:674–83.

13. Ezzat SM, Ezzat MI, Okba MM, et al. The hidden mechanism beyond ginger (Zingiber officianale Rosc.) potent in vivo and in vitro anti-inflammatory activity. J Ethnopharmacol 2018;214:113–23.

14. Webb S, editor. Nursing herbal medicine handbook. 3rd edition. Philadelphia: Lippincott Williams & Wilkins; 2006.

15. Rote NS. Infection. In: McCance KL, Huether SE, editors. Pathophysiology: the biologic basis for disease in adults and children. 8th edition. St. Louis (MO): Elsevier; 2019. p. 292–3.

16. Vasey C. Natural antibiotics and antivirals: 18 infection-fighting herbs and essential oils. Rochester (VT): Healing Arts Press; 2018. p. 1–208.

17. Fritz H. Cold and flu beyond: fending off viral invaders. Alive: Canada's Natural Health & Wellness Magazine 2019;443:17–22.

18. Zhu XY, Zeng YR. Garlic extract in prosthesis-related infections: a literature review. J Int Med Res 2020;48(4):1–10.

19. Denaro M, Smeriglio A, Barreca D, et al. Antiviral activity of plants and their isolated bioactive compounds: an update. Phytother Res 2020;34:742–68.

20. Shedoeva A, Leavesley D, Upton Z, et al. Wound healing and the use of medicinal plants. Evid Based Complement Alternat Med 2019;2019:1–30.

21. Mehreen A, Waheed M, Liaqat I, et al. Phytochemical, antimicrobial, and toxicological evaluation of traditional herbs used to treat sore throat. Biomed Res Int 2016;2016:1–9.

22. Mamatova AS, Korona-Glowniak I, Skalicka-Woaniak K, et al. Phytochemical composition of wormwood (Artemisia gmelinii) extracts in respect of their antimicrobial activity. BMC Complement Altern Med 2019;19(1):1–10.

23. Noronha M, Pawar V, Prajapati A, et al. A literature review on traditional herbal medicines for malaria. S Afr J Bot 2020;128:292–303.

24. Ashour RMS, Okba MM, Menze ET, et al. Eucalyptus sideroxylon bark anti-inflammatory potential, its UPLC-PDA-ESI-qTOF-MS profiling, and isolation of a new phloroglucinol. J Chromatogr Sci 2019;57(6):565–74.

25. Gunawardana SLA, Jayasuriya WJABN. Medicinally important herbal flowers in Sri Lanka. Evid Based Complement Alternat Med 2019;2019:1–18.

26. Fu B, Wu Q, Dang M, et al. Inhibition of pseudomonas aeruginosa biofilm formation by traditional Chinese medicinal herb Herba patriniae. Biomed Res Int 2017; 2017:9584703, 1-10.

27. Hickl J, Argyropoulou A, Sadavitsi ME, et al. Mediterranean herb extracts inhibit microbial growth of representative oral microorganisms and biofilm formation of Streptococcus mutans. PloS one 2018;13(12):e0207574.

28. Tsukatani T, Sakata F, Kuroda R, et al. Biofilm eradication activity of herb and spice extracts alone and in combination against oral and food-borne pathogenic bacteria. Curr Microbiol 2020;2020:1–10.

29. McCance KL, Grey TC, Rodway GW. Altered cellular and tissue biology: environmental agents. In: McCance KL, Huether SE, editors. Pathophysiology: the biologic basis for disease in adults and children. 8th edition. St. Louis (MO): Elsevier; 2019. p. 54–6.

30. Suleman M, Khan A, Baqi A, et al. Antioxidants, its role in preventing free radicals and infectious disease in human body. Pure and Applied Biology 2019;8(1): 380–8.

31. Dev SK, Choudhury PK, Srivastava R, et al. Antimicrobial, anti-inflammatory and wound healing activity of polyherbal formulation. Biomed Pharmacother 2019; 111:555–67.

32. Gulumian M, Yahaya ES, Steenkamp V. African herbal remedies with antioxidant activity: a potential resource base for wound treatment. Evid Based Complement Alternat Med 2018;2018:1–58.

33. Muluye RA, Bian Y, Alemu PN. Anti-inflammatory and antimicrobial effects of heat-clearing Chinese herbs: a current review. J Tradit Complement Med 2014; 4(2):93–8.

34. Xi S, Gong Y, editors. Herbs that clear heat. Essentials of Chinese material medica and medical formulas. London (United Kingdom): Academic Press Elsevier; 2017. p. 36–85.

35. Zhao T, Tang H, Xie L, et al. Scutellaria baicalensis georgi. (lamiaceae): a review of its traditional uses, botany, phytochemistry, pharmacology and toxicology. J Pharm Pharmacol 2019;71:1353–69.

36. Hu XY, Wu RH, Logue M, et al. Andrographis paniculata for symptomatic relief of acute respiratory tract infections in adults and children: a systematic review and meta-analysis. PloS one 2017;1–30. https://doi.org/10.1371/journal.pone. 0181780.

37. Wua J, Zhanga H, Hua B, et al. Immunopharmacology and inflammation Coptisine from Coptis chinensis inhibits production of inflammatory mediators in lipopolysaccharide-stimulated RAW 264.7 murine macrophage cells. Eur J Pharmacol 2016;780:106–14.

38. Hu C. Taraxacum: phytochemistry and health benefits. Chin Herbal Medicines 2018;10:353–61.

39. Guo Y, Lin L, Wang Y. Chemistry and pharmacology of the herb pair Flos lonicerae japonicae-Forythiae fructus. Chin Med 2015;10(1). https://doi.org/10. 1186/s13020-015-0044-y. Available at: https://link-gale-com.libdata.lib.ua.edu/ apps/doc/A541563744/AONE?u=tusc49521&sid=AONE&xid=7d9e52fd.

40. Li Y, Cai W, Weng X, et al. Lonicerae japonicae flos and Lonicerae flos: a systematic pharmacology review. Evid Based Complement Alternat Med 2015; 2015:1–16.

41. Huang Z, Pan X, Zhou J, et al. Chinese herbal medicine for acute upper respiratory tract infections and reproductive safety: a systematic review. Biosci Trends 2019;13(2):117–29.

42. Wang Z, Xia Q, Liu X, et al. Phytochemistry, pharmacology, quality control and future research of Forsythia suspense (Thunb.) vahl: a review. J Ethnopharmacol 2018;210:318–39.

43. Lu Y, Jiang Y, Ling L, et al. Beneficial effects of Houttuynia cordata polysaccharides on "two-hit" acute lung injury and endotoxic fever in rats associated with anti-complementary activities. Acta Pharm Sin B 2018;8(2):218–27.

44. Shingnaisui K, Dey T, Manna P, et al. Therapeutic potentials of Houttuynia cordata thunb. against inflammation and oxidative stress: a review. J Ethnopharmacol 2018;220:35–43.

45. Liao BL, Pan YJ, Zhang W, et al. Four natural compounds separated from Folium isatidis: crystal structures and antibacterial activity. Chem Biodivers 2018;15(7): 1–7 e1800152.

46. Suh SY, An WG. Systems pharmacological approach of Pulsatillae radix on treating Crohn's disease. Evid Based Complement Alternat Med 2017;1–21. https://doi.org/10.1155/2017/4198035.
47. Jeong YH, Oh YC, Cho WK, et al. Anti-inflammatory effects of Viola yedoensis and the application of cell extraction methods for investigating bioactive constituents in macrophages. BMC Complement Altern Med 2016;16:1–16.
48. Yu X, Ou L, Chen S, et al. Anti-inflammatory mechanism of Herba commelinae. Medicinal Plant 2016;7(1/2):32–4.
49. Ma X, Liu X, Feng J, et al. Fraxin alleviates LPS-induced ARDS by downregulating inflammatory responses and oxidative damages and reducing pulmonary vascular permeability. Inflammation 2019;42:1901–12.
50. Li X, Hu Q, Jiang S, et al. Flos chrysanthemi indici protects against hydroxyl-induced damages to DNA and MSCs via antioxidant mechanism. Journal of Saudi Chemical Society 2015;19(4):454–60.
51. Wu Y, Wang X, Xue J, et al. Plant phenolics extraction from flow chrysanthemi: response surface methodology based optimization and the correlation between extracts and free radical scavenging activity. J Food Sci 2017;82(11):2726–33.
52. Lin MY, Chiang SY, Li YZ, et al. Anti-tumor effect of *Radix paeoniae rubra* extract on mice bladder tumors using intravesical therapy. Oncol Lett 2016;12:904–10.
53. Xie P, Cui L, Shan Y, et al. Antithrombotic effect and mechanism of Radix paeoniae rubra. Biomed Res Int 2017;2017:1–9.
54. Ho LTF, Chan KKH, Chung VCH, et al. Highlights of traditional Chinese medicine frontline expert advice in the China national guideline for COVID-19. Eur J Integr Med 2020;36:1–5.

Traditional and Current Use of Ginseng

Amanda J. Flagg, PhD, RN, MSN/EdM, ACNS, CNE

KEYWORDS

- American ginseng • Asian ginseng • Siberian ginseng • Adaptogens • Ginsenosides

KEY POINTS

- There are many beneficial uses of all 3 types of ginseng.
- Use in children and pregnant women should be closely monitored by health care providers.
- There are few side effects; however, caution with impending surgical procedures and with uses of certain anticoagulants.

INTRODUCTION

Ginseng is a remarkable herb used medicinally over thousands of years in China, Japan, and Korea. The earliest known Chinese materia medica, *Shen Nong Ben Cao Jing,* addressed and categorized 365 herbs and recognized ginseng for its use in treating shortness of breath, fever, insomnia, forgetfulness, hemorrhage, and impotence.[1] These were just examples of uses for ginseng for many other health issues noted in this work. Shennong (the Divine Farmer) is credited as the author of this text, documenting herbs used approximately 5000 years earlier in China.[2,3] Not much else is known beyond this period.

During the past 300 years, ginseng has been cultivated in approximately 35 countries, to include the United States, and harvested for its specialized properties that are said to harness specific effects toward certain ailments and conditions in the human body.[4] Daniel Boone is credited for the early exploitation of wild-grown American ginseng while trail blazing during the 1780s period of early American history.[5] Since that time, this panacea has evolved into a supplement that holds numerous claims supporting benefits in conditions such as heart failure, respiratory diseases, circulatory issues, cancer, and dementia, to name a few.[1,2,6]

The key characteristics of this herb that nurses may find helpful when caring for patients using ginseng are addressed. The 3 most recognized types of ginseng are explored to include how each type works, general purported treatments regarding

Middle Tennessee State University (MTSU) School of Nursing, MTSU Box 81, Murfreesboro, TN 37132, USA
E-mail address: amanda.flagg@mtsu.edu

Nurs Clin N Am 56 (2021) 109–121
https://doi.org/10.1016/j.cnur.2020.10.011
0029-6465/21/© 2020 Elsevier Inc. All rights reserved.

specific conditions and disease states, beneficial effects on the body, major interactions with other medications and herbs, side effects, contraindications, and dosage. Please note that the use of any type or form of ginseng is not recommended for pediatric patients unless closely monitored by a physician. Therefore, this article only addresses use of ginseng in adults. To begin to understand the broad claims of why ginseng is reported to be so effective for a vast many conditions and disease states requires the understanding of its characterization as an adaptogen.

DEFINING ADAPTOGENS

Adaptogens come from natural substances that are nonspecific in nature but aid the human body by resisting the effects of stressful conditions that can affect the immune, neurologic, and endocrine systems.[7] Traditional Chinese medicine recognized the value of ginseng in aiding the human body by deflecting these types of stresses they felt were causes of illness and disruptions in the harmony of an individuals' health.[1–3] The term and concept "adaptogen" was proposed by a Russian scientist, N. Lazarev in 1940. Other scientists expanded the concept of adaptogens that included categorizations, mechanisms of actions, and useful applications.[7] Traditional uses of ginseng have become the springboard for current and future uses of ginseng in the form of tonics and oral preparations and as adaptogens in the treatment of many conditions described 5000 years earlier. So, what are the types of ginseng and how are each used in current times?

DISCUSSION
Types of Ginseng

Ginseng's root resembles a human being with several "arms and legs." It is the root that contains properties called ginsenosides that are major sources of most preparations. Roots come from plants that are typically 5 years of age and older. Ginsenosides are the active chemicals similar in nature to steroids, making ginseng highly valued by a multitude of consumers.[4] The type of ginseng, ginsenosides, and preparation of the herbs produce properties influencing the effects that ginseng has on certain diseases and conditions.

Three types of ginseng include Panax ginseng (Asian, Korean, or Red ginseng); Panax quinquefolis, which is also known as American ginseng; and Siberian ginseng or Eleutherococcus senticosus[8] (**Table 1**). The growth and harvesting of American ginseng is described because its export to many countries has become world-wide and recognized as a source of many over-the-counter ginseng products.

Three Methods of Growing American Ginseng

American ginseng is harvested from 3 distinct sources: (1) wild ginseng, specifically found in forests of Northeastern United States and Canada, (2) wild-simulated ginseng where seeds are planted in woods that provide similar shade and soil to where wild ginseng grows but no fertilizer or other forms of artificial herbicides are used, and (3) field-cultivated ginseng, where artificial shade is provided over seeds planted in raised beds. Wild ginseng and wild-simulated ginseng are reported to produce similar effects in terms of quality of the root, whereas field-cultivated ginseng tends to be of lower quality but higher volume of product.[10,11]

Since 1975, the Convention on International Trade in Endangered Species of Wild Fauna and Flora in the United States has placed ginseng on its protective list with 400 other plants. Strict regulations around the harvesting of wild sources of ginseng root include such restrictions as outlined: (1) there needs to be at least 3 leaves present

Table 1
General effects of ginsenosides and/or eleutherosides for each type of ginseng

Type of Ginseng	Location of Growth	General Effects
American ginseng or Panax quinquefolis	North America and Canada	Calming effect Increased neurocognitive function Anticancer properties Decreased blood pressure Decreased stress Decreased blood glucose Decreased free radicals
Asian ginseng or Panax ginseng	Asia (to include China, Korea, and Japan)	Increased physical stamina Increased mental concentration Increased immunity Decreased erectile dysfunction Increased sexual performance
Siberian ginseng or Eleutherococcus Senticosus = (active chemicals are known as eleutherosides)	Most parts of Russia	Increased T-cell production Decreased lengths and severity of colds Increased energy Increased cognitive function Increased physical performance

Data from Refs.[4,6–9]

(making the plant at least 5 years in age), (2) 19 states within the United States are regulated under the Convention on International Trade in Endangered Species of Wild Fauna and Flora, and (3) the harvesting of wild ginseng can only take place during designated harvest seasons. Harvesting of field cultivated ginseng does not fall under the Convention on International Trade in Endangered Species of Wild Fauna and Flora's direction.[4]

How Ginseng Is Harvested

Television shows, like the *Appalachian Outlaws* and *Smoky Mountain Gold,* share the fact that cultivating ginseng is not only lucrative, but carries stiff penalties for those who are illegally harvesting wild ginseng. Only landowners can give permission for harvesting wild grown ginseng on their property, yet poachers continue to illegally hunt and harvest ginseng roots regardless of penalties imposed.[12,13]

Values of ginseng root continue to increase annually. Dried roots sell for $ 500 to $1000, depending on the age, condition, and source of the roots. Families who have been harvesting American ginseng recognize that conservation efforts of preserving wild ginseng is a constant challenge. For example, families in Appalachia have relied heavily on harvesting and selling American ginseng for many generations. With increasing private land ownership and government control of national forestry, these families often resort to risking their lives when seeking the product that literally kept their families from starvation. Therefore, farming ginseng has become a trade that is not currently only advantageous to buyers here in the United States, but also abroad, specifically Asia, where surprisingly several tons of ginseng are exported annually.[4,12,13]

Preparations

Ginseng, no matter the type, is distributed for use in all forms. Preparations specifically for American ginseng (dried) is available for use in the following forms: powders, water, combinations with other elements, capsules, alcohol herbs, and formulas.

Tablets and Extracts

Other forms of American ginseng are available as a standard extract, fresh or dried root, tincture, or a type of fluid extract. Additionally, American ginseng is known to be slightly less potent regardless of preparation than Asian ginseng. **Table 2** outlines common sources of ginseng by different forms of ingestion.[14]

CURRENT EVIDENCE

There are so many claims regarding healing properties of any kind of ginseng to a vast and diverse number of human diseases and conditions. Only those conditions and disease states that have been studied using some form of research will be acknowledged by body system, disease or condition, and the influence of ginseng to the specific disease process or processes.

Cardiovascular System

American and Asian ginseng have been shown to improve cardiac function through animal models and humans by researching specific actions of ginseng and related ginsenosides, specifically Rb_1, Rg_1, Rg_3, Re, and Rd, which are the most studied in current literature to date. Major causes of cardiovascular risk include cigarette smoking, increased low-density lipoprotein cholesterol, decreased high-density lipoprotein cholesterol, hypertension, and diabetes. **Table 3** outlines studied effects of ginseng to conditions related to the cardiovascular system.[15–19]

Inversely, during exercise ginseng has been shown to significantly increase heart rate and blood pressure with exercise along with increased oxygen levels to active muscle groups. Participants in these studies claimed that ginseng use enhanced their endurance and recovery times after exercise.[15]

Digestive System

Two studies found Asian ginseng to be effective in the provision of improving gut microbiota when treating ulcerative colitis. Asian ginseng was effective in the relief of symptoms of ulcerative colitis by promoting probiotic growth, which also provided protection from *Staphylococcus aureus* and *Salmonella*. More studies are needed to fully understand how Asian ginseng can be used in controlling and possibly preventing ulcerative colitis symptoms and other similar types of conditions.[20–22]

Musculoskeletal System

American, Asian, and Siberian ginseng are reported as being helpful in the treatment of pain relief and inflammation of joints; however, there are no studies that support its direct effect as a treatment for specific conditions of the musculoskeletal system.[23]

Table 2
Common preparations of American, Asian, and Siberian ginseng

Type of Ginseng	Preparation	Product
American ginseng	Boiled, dried, fresh	Soups, teas, tonics Capsules, powders, slices of raw root (tastes like bitter radishes)
Asian ginseng	Dried, fermented, steamed	Root powder, capsules, extracts, oils
Siberian ginseng	Dried, steamed	Infusions and seasonings

Table 3
Effects of ginseng on the cardiovascular system

Condition/Disease	Type of Ginseng	Affect	Risk
Coronary artery diagnosis	American/Asian	Multiple protective Affects	Cardiotoxic potential
Myocardial ischemia	American/Asian	Increased exercise tolerance and improved electrocardiographic studies	
Heart failure	American/Asian	Decreased presence of ascites	–
Cardiac contractility	American/Asian	Decreased ventricular hypertrophy	
Calcium channel affects	American/Asian	Inhibition of mitochondria swelling Increased energy metabolism Decreased heart rate	

Endocrine System

Many claims have been made throughout the history of ginseng regarding its' effects on the endocrine system. Multiple studies show promising findings. With the advancement of technology aiding in understanding mechanisms of these herbs, **Table 3** outlines repetitive findings of the effects of mostly Asian ginseng to conditions under the influence of the endocrine system[24–30] (**Table 4**).

Integumentary System

Fermented Asian ginseng is used to whiten skin, decreases wrinkles, protect against ultraviolet radiation–induced skin damage, and increase regeneration of hyaluronic acid, a key component in the preservation and antiaging effects of skin. Research studies are well-supported by bench science and hold promising predictions based on the specific roles certain ginsenosides play in addition to claims made in antiaging properties of human skin. Animal models are holding promising findings regarding ginseng's role in the healing of wounds and other types of skin disorders.[31,32]

Neurologic System

Substantial studies have been conducted relating the effects of Asian ginseng to possible treatment options of several neurologic conditions. A major find reflects

Table 4
Effects of ginseng on the endocrine system

Condition/Disease	Type of Ginseng	Affect	Additional Note
Type II diabetes	American/Asian	Stabilization of glucose	Not as effective with
Erectile dysfunction	Asian	levels with increased	type I diabetes –
Male fertility	Asian	lipid metabolism	potential for weight loss
Menopause	American/Asia	Increased performance	exists
Stress	Asian	Increased spermatogenesis	Asian is the preferred type
		Decreased symptoms	Mixed reviews on
		Stabilizing effect on	effectiveness
		the sympathetic	
		nervous system and	
		central nervous system	

the protective properties certain ginsenosides exhibit to neurons in the body. Another finding demonstrates how ginsenoside Rg1 produces an antidepressant effect that equates to the use of the medication, imipramine, frequently prescribed for depression in adult patients. Additionally, panaxatriol saponins, fruits of Asian ginseng, interact with the neurotransmitter, serotonin. Platelets contain upwards of 99% of serotonin at injury sites of vascular structures. Imbalances of this neurotransmitter may involve coronary heart disease and depression through impaired platelet function and mental status. **Table 5** outlines studies about additional interactions ginseng may display on the human neurologic system.[33–46]

Cognition and Mood

Asian ginseng has been noted to improve cognition levels not only in individuals with mild cognitive impairments, but also in individuals diagnosed with Alzheimer's disease. Volunteers with no demonstrable cognitive difficulties were reported to sharpen their cognition and memory with the use of a 1-time dose of American ginseng. Studies continue to explore not only how this is done, but how moods are also enhanced with those patients diagnosed with depression and anxiety.[47–52]

Other Conditions Affecting Body Systems

Ginseng has a long association with treatments pertaining to cancer, immunity, colds and flu, and inflammatory effects. **Table 6** outlines the interactions of these treatments with positively associated types of ginseng to the condition or disease. Results of most studies regarding effects to these conditions have been positive regarding action of certain ginsenosides in the use of mice models. More research with human subjects is needed to ascertain safety and possible drug interactions with conventional treatments.[53–64]

Side Effects

It is important to remember that not all sources of ginseng sold over the counter, no matter the type, are of equal quality. Owing to lack of standardization, some products professing to be a type of ginseng or advertising the presence of certain ginsenosides may not have any form of ginseng or any other kind of herb.[65] Many over-the-counter medications may include such substances as dangerous heavy metals or properties that have little to no significant effects attributed to ginseng. Therefore, any side effect experienced by the consumer will s careful exploration on the part of both the consumer and health care provider.

   The good news is that there are very few instances of reportable side effects experienced by consumers of ginseng. Rare instances are continually studied and are more fully understood with increasing interest separating myth from science. Most studies involved on potential side effects of ginseng include Asian ginseng owing to its more

Table 5
Effects of ginseng on the neurologic system

Condition/Disease	Type of Ginseng	Affect	Risk
Stroke (ischemic)	Asian	Neuroprotective affects	More studies needed
Seizures	Asian	Anticonvulsant properties – ginsenosides Rb1 and 3	
Parkinson's disease	Asian		
Alzheimer's disease	Asian	Neuroprotective affects	
Huntington's disease	Asian		
Spinal cord injury	Asian		
Attention Deficit Disorder	Asian		

Table 6 Common interactions of categories of medications with American ginseng		
Medication Type	**Possible Interaction**	**Level of Risk**
Antidiabetic	Decreased blood glucose level	Moderate risk based on type of diabetes and glucose control
Anticoagulant	Decreased effect of warfarin Caution with use of nonsteroidal anti-inflammatory drugs, aspirin, other anticoagulants	Moderate risk increased bruising/bleeding with wounds and other types of injuries
Monoamine oxidase inhibitors	May exaggerate effects of monoamine oxidase inhibitors in treatment of depression	Mild to moderate risk Manic episodes could be triggered, although rarely documented

robust nature when compared with that of American ginseng. Regardless of the type of ginseng, the most reported side effects are as follows[6,8,66]:

- Diarrhea
- Insomnia
- Headache
- Increased heart rate
- Increased or decreased blood pressure
- Possible breast tenderness and vaginal bleeding

When combined with substances containing caffeine, increased jitteriness with possible increased feelings of uneasiness and insomnia have been known to occur. Inversely, when taken with alcohol, reports of Asian ginseng suggest that there is an enhanced effect that increases the metabolism and breakdown of alcohol ingested.[67] As with any form of herb or medication along with side effects, there are contraindications and interactions with other medications to consider.

Caution with Use

There are situations along with many interactions to contemplate when considering the use of ginseng as either a dietary supplement, enhancer of an effect, or as a sole form of treatment. **Tables 6** and **7** tables provide outlines of the more common interactions found in the literature based on findings from 2015 to 2020. Medication interactions are not inclusive, but the more commonly studied interactions are outlined in **Tables 6** and **7** for American and Asian ginseng.[68–70]

One additional contraindication worth considering is the use of any type of ginseng before a surgical procedure. Owing to the potential effects of prolonging prothrombin time, the patient may also suffer from hypoglycemia, particularly when mandatory fasting is required. Education of patients who report the use and ingestion of ginseng should be advised to withhold ginseng from 24 hours to upwards of 7 days before the procedure.[71,72]

How Much Is Too Much?

Dosing of ginseng depends on the type and preparation of the ginseng product. In general terms recommended dosage for the following conditions when Asian ginseng is used as examples are:

Table 7
Common interactions of categories of medications with Asian ginseng

Medication Type	Possible Interaction	Level of Risk
Antihypertensives	Possible decreased of medication effectiveness	Low with very little effect on essential or "white coat" hypertension Caution: calcium channel blockers, statins
Antiplatelet/antithrombotic	Possible increased effect of medication	Low level
Central nervous system stimulants	Possible increased effect	Low level
Human immunodeficiency virus integrase inhibitors	May increased adverse effects	Low level
Antidiabetic	Decreased blood glucose levels	Low to Moderate Level
Monoamine oxidase inhibitors	Increased side effects such as headache, tremors, insomnia	Contraindicated

Data from Potential herb-drug interactions for commonly used herbs (ginseng). 2020. Available at standardprocess.com/MediHerb-Document-Library/Catalog-Files/herb-drug-interaction-chart.pdf.

- Chronic obstructive pulmonary disease: 100 mg to 6 g 3 times a day
- Memory/cognition: 200 mg to 400 mg/d
- Erectile dysfunction: 1400 mg to 2700 mg in 2 to 3 divided doses daily
- Flu: before taking a flu vaccine and 8 weeks after, up to 1 g/d
- Fatigue: 250 mg twice daily

These examples are by no means prescriptive. They are based on prior use and proclaimed effectiveness of individuals who have used ginseng accordingly for a period of 3 months.

It is highly recommended that guidance from a health care provider be sought before taking ginseng with specific intentions in mind.[73,74]

SUMMARY

Ginseng was explored in terms of history, type, preparations, effects on body systems, side effects, interactions with other forms of medications, and general dosing guidelines. Centuries have passed since the documentation of early uses of ginseng. The consensus of many practitioners of medicine still holds the belief that this most remarkable herb is indeed a panacea for an extraordinary number of disease states. Evidence shows that we are still in the early stages of understanding just how remarkable this herb is. As science continues to evolve, so will the understanding of the value of ginseng to present day and future use.

CLINICS CARE POINTS

- Always consult a health care provider before consuming ginseng of any kind especially if other forms of medication are being used.
- Different types of ginseng will illicit different effects in the human body.
- While side effects of differing types of ginseng are rare, further research is needed to substantiate specific reactions.
- One known contraindication is the use of ginseng prior to and after a surgical procedure due to potential effects of prolonged prothrombin time and hypoglycemia.

- Dosages of ginseng will vary based on the type of ginseng consumed.

DISCLOSURE

This author has nothing to disclose.

REFERENCES

1. Unschuld PU, Andrews B. Traditional Chinese medicine. New York (NY): Columbia University Press; 2018. Available at: https://ebookcentral.proquest.com/lib/[SITE_ID]/detail.action?docID=5276126.

2. Xiang Y, Shang H, Gao X, et al. A comparison of the ancient use of ginseng in traditional Chinese medicine with modern pharmacological experiments and clinical trials. Phytother Res 2008;22(7):851–8. Available at: https://onlinelibrary.wiley.com/doi/abs/10.1002/ptr.2384.

3. Slazinski L. History of ginseng. JAMA 1979;242(7):616.

4. U.S. Fish & Wildlife Service. International Affairs. American ginseng. Available at: www.fws.gov/international Web site. fws.gov/international/plants/american-ginseng.html. Accessed May 23, 2020.

5. Halstead R. Daniel Boone and ginseng. 1995.Audio. Available at: https://www.loc.gov/item/cmns001802/. Accessed May 23, 2020.

6. Davis MPBB. Ginseng: a qualitative review of benefits for palliative clinicians. Am J Hosp Palliat care 2019;36(7):630–59.

7. Liao L, He Y, Li L, et al. A preliminary review of studies on adaptogens: comparison of their bioactivity in TCM with that of ginseng-like herbs used worldwide. Chin Med 2018;13(1):57. Available at: https://www.ncbi.nlm.nih.gov/pubmed/30479654.

8. Keville K. Ginseng: getting to the root of this versatile herb. Better Nutrition 2001;63(5):48–52. Available at: http://search.ebscohost.com/login.aspx?direct=true&db=ccm&AN=106979126&site=ehost-live&scope=site. Accessed November 11, 2020.

9. Lee SM, Bae B, Park H, et al. Characterization of Korean red ginseng (panax ginseng): history, preparation method, and chemical composition. J Ginseng Res 2015;39(4):384–91.

10. Staff resources MS. American ginseng. mountsiani.org Web site. 2020. Available at. mountsiani.org/health-library/herb/American-ginseng. Accessed May 28, 2020.

11. Tsai E. American ginseng pharm. americanginsengpharm.com Web site. 2016. Available at. americanginsengpharm.com/post/2016/02/17/the-difference-between-wild-simulated ginseng-with cultivated-ginseng. Accessed May 25, 2020.

12. Associated Press. New reality show focuses on West Virginia ginseng business. Sacramento. 2013. Available at. cbslocal.com/2013/12/25/new-reality-show-focuses-on-west-virginia-ginseng-business/. Accessed May 20, 2020.

13. Board G. Ginseng reality TV: cultivating conservation or encouraging extinction?/ 0 Web site. 2014. Available at. wvpublic.org/post/ginseng-reality-tv-cultivating-conservation-or-encouraging-extinction#stream. Accessed May 20, 2020.

14. Dharmananda S. The nature of ginseng: traditional use, modern research, and the question of dosage. HerbalGram 2002;54:34–51. American Botanical Council.

15. Zahren Sa, Marandi SMZ. The effect of ginseng supplement on heart rate, systolic and diastolic blood pressure to resistance training in trained males. Artery Res 2016;(15):6–11.

16. Kim J. Pharmacological and medical applications of panax ginseng and ginsenosides: a review for use in cardiovascular diseases. J Ginseng Res 2017;42(3): 264–9.

17. Komishon AM, Shishtar E, Ha V, et al. The effect of ginseng (genus panax) on blood pressure: a systematic review and meta-analysis of randomized controlled clinical trials. J Hum Hypertens 2016;30(10):619–26. Available at. https://ezproxy.mtsu.edu/login?url=http://search.ebscohost.com/login.aspx?direct=true&db=mnh&AN=27074879&site=ehost-live&scope=site.

18. Wang M, Lei Y. Time-effect relationship of extracts from ginseng, notoginseng and chuanxiong on vascular endothelial cells senescence. Chin J Integr Med 2014; 20(10):758–63. Available at. https://ezproxy.mtsu.edu/login?url=http://search.ebscohost.com/login.aspx?direct=true&db=ccm&AN=103903894&site=ehost-live&scope=site.

19. Zheng S, Wu H, Wu D. Roles and mechanisms of ginseng in protecting heart. Chin J Integr Med 2012;18(7):548–55. Available at. http://search.ebscohost.com/lo gin.aspx?direct=true&db=ccm&AN=104475496&site=ehost-live&scope=site.

20. Guo M, Ding S, Hao C, et al. s. Red ginseng and semen coicis can improve the structure of gut microbiota and relieve the symptoms of ulcerative colitis. J Ethnopharmacol 2015;162:7–13.

21. Mehendale S, Aung H, Wang A, et al. North American ginseng berry extract and ginsenoside. Ginseng Ontario Web site. Available at. http://ginsengontario.com/about/health-benefitd/digestie-system/. Accessed May 28, 2020.

22. Oyagi A, Kenjirou O, Kakino M, et al. Protective effects of a gastrointestinal agent containing Korean red ginseng on gastric ulcer models in mice. BMC Complement Altern Med 2010;10(45). https://doi.org/10.1186/1472-6882-10-45.

23. Pumpa KL, Fallon KE, Papalia S, Bensoussan A. Tienchi Ginseng for the treatment and prevention of delayed onset muscle soreness and muscle damage in well-trained athletes: a double-blind randomised controlled trial....13th annual symposium on complementary health care, 12th-14th December, 2006, University of Exeter, UK. Focus on Alternative & Complementary Therapies. 2006; 11:37-38. Available at. http://search.ebscohost.com.ezprox. Accessed June 9, 2020.

24. Zhao Y, Zheng j, Yu Y, et al. Panax notoginseng Saponins Regulate Macrophage Polarization under hyperglycemic condition via NF-kB Signaling Pathway. Biomed Res Int 2018;2018:1–8.

25. Oh MR, Park SH, Kim SY, et al. Does fermented red ginseng (Panax ginseng) influence glucose metabolism in humans? Focus on Alternative & Complementary Therapies 2015;20(1):40. https://doi.org/10.1111/fct.12150.

26. Irani M, Sardassht FG, Ghazanfarpour M, et al. Systematic overview of reviews on the efficacy of complementary and alternative medicine in erectile dysfunction. Journal of Midwifery & Reproductive Health 2018;6(4):1476–85. https://doi.org/10.22038/jmrh.2018.29476.1318.

27. Borelli F, Colalto C, Delfino DV, et al. Herbal dietary supplements for erectile dysfunction: a systematic review and meta-analysis. Drugs 2018;78(6):643–73.

28. Kiefer D. Red ginseng and menopause. Integrative Medicine Alert 2013;16(3): 34–5. Available at: http://search.ebscohost.com.ezproxy.mtsu.edu/login.aspx?direct=true&db=ccm&AN=85930391&site=ehost-live&scope=site. Accessed November 11, 2020.

29. Baek JH, Heo J, Fava M, et al. Effect of Korean red ginseng in individuals exposed to high stress levels: a 6-week, double-blind, randomized, placebo-controlled trial. J Ginseng Res 2019;43(3):402–7. Available at. http://www.sciencedirect.com/science/article/pii/S1226845317302749.

30. Lee SRD. Effects of ginseng on stress-related depression, anxiety, and the hypothalamic-pituitary-adrenal axis. J Ginseng Res 2017;41(4):589–94.

31. Park S, Daily JW, Lee J. Can topical use of ginseng or ginsenosides accelerate wound healing? J Med Food 2018;21(11):1075–6.

32. Lee G, Park K, Namgoong S, et al. Effects of Panax ginseng extract on human dermal fibroblast proliferation and collagen synthesis. Int Wound J 2016;13:42–6.

33. Seyed FN, Sureda A, Habtemariam S, et al. Ginsenoside rd and ischemic stroke; a short review of literatures. J Ginseng Res 2015;39(4):299–303.

34. Rasttogi V, Santiago-Moreno J, Dore S. Ginseng: a promising neuroprotective strategy in stroke. Front Cell Neurosci 2014;8:457.

35. Stringer JL. Ginseng and other herbal treatments for epilepsy. St Louis (MO): Elsevier Inc; 2017. https://doi.org/10.1016/B978-0-12-809324-5.00245-5.

36. Liu Wei, Ge T, Pan Z, et al. The effects of herbal medicine on epilepsy. Oncotarget 2017;8(29):48385–97.

37. Razgonova MP, Veselov VV, Zakharenko AM, et al. Panax ginseng components and the pathogenesis of Alzheimer's disease (review). Mol Med Rep 2019;19(4):2975–98. Available at: http://search.ebscohost.com/login.aspx?direct=true&db=mnh&AN=30816465&site=ehost-live&scope=site.

38. Wu JG, Wang YY, Zhang ZL, et al. Herbal medicine in the treatment of Alzheimer's disease. Chin J Integr Med 2015;21(2):102–7.

39. Zhu P, Samukawa K, Fujita H, et al. Oral administration of red ginseng extract promotes neurorestoration after compressive spinal cord injury in rats. Evid Based Complement Alternat Med 2017;2017:10.

40. Cho I. Effects of panax ginseng in neurodegenerative diseases. J Ginseng Res 2012;36(4):342–53. Available at: https://www.ncbi.nlm.nih.gov/pubmed/23717136.

41. Lee J, Lee A, Kim J, et al. Effect of omega-3 and Korean red ginseng on children with attention deficit hyperactivity disorder: an open-label pilot study. Clin Psychopharmacol Neurosci 2020;18(1):75–80. Available at: https://www.ncbi.nlm.nih.gov/pubmed/31958908.

42. Sung MN, Choi JH, Choi SH, et al. Ginseng gintonin alleviates neurological symptoms in the G93A-SOD1 transgenic mouse model of amyotrophic lateral sclerosis through lysophosphatidic acid 1 receptor. J Ginseng Res 2020;0. https://doi.org/10.1016/j.jgr.2020.04.002.

43. Hou W, Wang Y, Zheng P, et al. Effects of ginseng on neurological disorders. Front Cell Neurosci 2020;14. https://doi.org/10.3389/fncel.2020.00055.

44. Rajabian A, Rameshrad M, Hosseinzadeh H. Therapeutic potential of panax ginseng and its constituents, ginsenosides and gintonin, in neurological and neurodegenerative disorders: a patent review. Expert Opin Ther Pat 2019;29(1):55–72.

45. Rokot NT, Kairupan, Cheng KT, et al. A role of ginseng and its constituents in the treatment of central nervous system disorders. Evid Based Complement Alternat Med 2016;2016:2614742.

46. Niederhofer H. Panax ginseng may improve some symptoms of attention-deficit hyperactivity disorder. J Diet Suppl 2009;6(1):22–7. Available at: https://ezproxy.mtsu.edu/login?url=http://search.ebscohost.com/login.aspx?direct=true&db=mnh&AN=22435351&site=ehost-live&scope=site.

47. Park KC, Jin H, Zheng R, et al. Cognition enhancing effect of panax ginseng in Korean volunteers with mild cognitive impairment: a randomized, double-blind, placebo-controlled clinical trial. Transl Clin Pharmacol 2019;27(3):92–7.

48. Kennedy DO. Phytochemicals for improving aspects of cognitive function and psychological state potentially relevant to sports performance. Sports Med 2019;49(Suppl 1):S39–58.

49. Carmichael OT, Pillai S, Shankapal P, et al. A combination of essential fatty acids, panax ginseng extract, and green tea catechins modifies brain fMRI signals in healthy older adults. J Nutr Health Aging 2018;22(7):837–46. Available at: https://ezproxy.mtsu.edu/login?url=http://search.ebscohost.com/login.aspx?direct=true&db=ccm&AN=130795790&site=ehost-live&scope=site.

50. Ossoukhova A, Owen L, Savage K, et al. Improved working memory performance following administration of a single dose of american ginseng (panax quinquefolius L.) to healthy middle-age adults. Hum Psychopharmacol 2015;30(2):108–22. Available at: https://ezproxy.mtsu.edu/login?url=http://search.ebscohost.com/login.aspx?direct=true&db=mnh&AN=25778987&site=ehost-live&scope=site.

51. Al RJ, Kennedy DO, Scholey AB. Effects of panax ginseng, consumed with and without glucose, on blood glucose levels and cognitive performance during sustained 'mentally demanding' tasks. J Psychopharmacol 2006;20(6):771–81. Available at: https://www-ncbi-nlm-nih-gov.ezproxy.mtsu.edu/pubmed/16401645. Accessed Feb 27, 2020.

52. Niederhofer H. First preliminary results with an observation of panax ginseng treatment in patients with autistic disorder. J Diet Suppl 2009;6(4):342–6. Available at: www.inforaworld.com/WIDS.

53. Choi SH, Yan KJ, Lee DS. Effects of complementary combination therapy of Korean red ginseng and antiviral agents in chronic hepatitis B. J Altern Complement Med 2016;22(12):964–9.

54. Lucius K. Diet, botanical medicine, and nutraceuticals for chronic kidney disease. Alternative and Complementary Therapies 2019;25(6):312–9. https://doi.org/10.1089/act.2019.29250.klu.

55. Shergis JL, Di YM, Zhang AL, et al. Therapeutic potential of panax ginseng and ginsenosides in the treatment of chronic obstructive pulmonary disease. Complement Ther Med 2014;22:944–53.

56. Li T, Sun W, Dong X, et al. Total ginsenosides of Chinese ginseng induces cell cycle arrest and apoptosis colorectal carcinoma HT-29 cells. Oncol Lett 2018;16:4640–8.

57. Hsu WL, Tsai YT, Wu CT, et al. The prescription pattern of Chinese herbal products containing ginseng among tamoxifen-treated female breast cancer Taiwan: a population-based study. Evid Based Complement Alternat Med 2015;1–11. https://doi.org/10.1155/2015/385204.

58. Pourmohamadi K, Ahmadzadeh A, Latifi M. Investigating the effects of oral ginseng on the cancer-related fatigue and quality of life in patients with non-metastatic cancer. Int J Hematol Oncol Stem Cell Res 2018;12(4):312–6. Available at: ijhoscr.turns.ac.ir.

59. Ahuja A, Ki JH, Kim JH, et al. Functional role of ginseng-derived compounds in cancer. J Ginseng Res 2018;42:248–54.

60. Xiao J, Chen D, Lin X, et al. Screening of drug metabolizing enzymes for the ginsenoside compound K in vitro: an efficient anti-cancer substance originating from panax ginseng. PLoS One 2016;11(2):e0147183. Available at: https://ezproxy.mtsu.edu/login?url=http://search.ebscohost.com/login.aspx?direct=true&db=mnh&AN=26845774&site=ehost-live&scope=site.

61. Seida JK, Durec T, Kuhle S. North American (panax quinquefolius) and Asian ginseng (panax ginseng) preparations for prevention of the common cold in healthy adults: a systematic review. Evid Based Complement Alternat Med 2011;2011:282151. https://doi.org/10.1093/ecam/nep068. Available at: https://ezproxy.mtsu.edu/login?url=https://search.proquest.com/docview/2060808756?accountid=4886.

62. North American (panax quinquefolius) and Asian ginseng (panax ginseng) preparations for prevention of the common cold in healthy adults: a systematic review - ProQuest. Available at: https://search-proquest-com.ezproxy.mtsu.edu/docview/2060808756/fulltextPDF/85E771CCC4BE4C26PQ/1?accountid=4886. Accessed Feb 27, 2020.

63. Abdelfattah-Hassan A, Shalaby SI, Khater SI, et al. Panax ginseng is superior to vitamin E as a hepatoprotector against cyclophosphamide-induced liver damage. Complement Ther Med 2019;46:95–102. Available at: https://search.proquest.com/docview/2287407406?accountid=4886.

64. Jin Y, Cui R, Zhao L, et al. Mechanisms of panax ginseng action as an antidepressant. Cell Prolif 2019;52(6):e12696. Available at: https://ezproxy.mtsu.edu/login?url=http://search.ebscohost.com/login.aspx?direct=true&db=mnh&AN=31599060&site=ehost-live&scope=site.

65. Sachan AK, Vishnoi G, Kumar R. Need of standardization of herbal medicines in modern era. International Journal of Phytomedicine 2016;8(3):300. https://doi.org/10.5138/09750185.1847.

66. Mancuso C, Santangelo R. Panax ginseng and panax quinquefolius: from pharmacology to toxicology. Food Chem Toxicol 2017;107:362–72. Available at: http://www.sciencedirect.com.ezproxy.mtsu.edu/science/article/pii/S0278691517303915.

67. Lee MH, Kwak JH, Jeon G, et al. Red ginseng relieves the effects of alcohol consumption and hangover symptoms in healthy men: a randomized crossover study. Food Funct 2014;5(3):528–34.

68. Ashner GN, Corbett AH, Hawke RL. Common herbal dietary supplement-drug interactions. Am Fam Physician 2017;96(2):101–7.

69. Singh A, Zhao K. Herb-drug interactions of commonly used Chinese medicinal herbs. Int Rev Neurobiol 2017;135:197–232. Available at: https://www.ncbi.nlm.nih.gov/pubmed/28807159.

70. Potential herb-drug interactions for commonly used herbs (ginseng). 2020. Available at: standardprocess.com/MediHerb-Document-Library/Catalog-Files/herb-drug-interaction-chart.pdf. Accessed May 11, 2020.

71. Powell A. Effect of herbal medicines during surgery. Plast Surg Nurs 2017;99. https://doi.org/10.1097/psn.0000000000000191.

72. Lee S, Ahn Y, Ahn S, et al. Interaction between warfarin and panax ginseng in ischemic stroke patients. J Altern Complement Med 2008;14(6):715–21. Available at: https://ezproxy.mtsu.edu/login?url=http://search.ebscohost.com/login.aspx?direct=true&db=ccm&AN=105681890&site=ehost-live&scope=site.

73. Baldaia L. Panax and pharmaceuticals: adding an herb to enhance medical treatment. Am J Nurse Pract 2005;9(9):9–17. Available at: http://search.ebscohost.com/login.aspx?direct=true&db=ccm&AN=106543249&site=ehost-live&scope=site.

74. Ginseng P. dosing. 2019. Available at: webmd.com/vitamins/ai/ingredientmoo-1000/panax-ginseng. Accessed June 9, 2020.

Herbal Medications Used to Ameliorate Cardiac Conditions

Maria A. Revell, PhD, MSN, RN, COI[a],*,
Marcia A. Pugh, DNP, MSN, MBA, HCM, RN[b]

KEYWORDS

- Cardiovascular disease • Herbs • Ginsenoside • Catechin • Silybum

KEY POINTS

- In the United States, herbal medications are regulated by the US Food and Drug Administration.
- Herbs may be used by clients exclusively for cardiovascular disease or in combination with conventional medications.
- Although there is research related to specific herbs, there is also much more to learn relative to their effect on the human body and specifically the cardiovascular system.
- It is important for the care provider to discuss possible benefits and side effects that may occur taking herbs in isolation or in combination with cardiovascular prescription medications.

INTRODUCTION

Herbs have been used for centuries to treat various diseases inclusive of cardiovascular disease. Herbs may be used by clients exclusively for disease or in combination with conventional medications. Unlike conventional medications, the efficacy of herbal use in the treatment of cardiovascular disease is not often research based. The purpose of this article is not to promote the use of herbs over other forms of treatment, but to make the health care provider aware of certain herbs and their potential use by clients as well as their impact on the cardiovascular system. It is important for the advanced practice nurse to collect information related to herb use during history retrieval. It is also important for the care provider to discuss the possible benefits as well as side effects that may occur taking herbs in isolation or in combination with cardiovascular prescription medications.

[a] Tennessee State University, School of Nursing, 3500 John A. Merritt Boulevard, Campus Box 9590, Nashville, TN 37209, USA; [b] Greene County Health System, 509 Wilson Avenue, Eutaw, AL 35462, USA
* Corresponding author. 214 Jon Paul Court, Murfreesboro, TN 37128.
E-mail address: mrevell1@tnstate.edu

Nurs Clin N Am 56 (2021) 123–136
https://doi.org/10.1016/j.cnur.2020.10.009
0029-6465/21/© 2020 Elsevier Inc. All rights reserved.
nursing.theclinics.com

USE OF HERBS IN THE UNITED STATES AND OTHER COUNTRIES

The reported use of herbs worldwide is as high as 80%. The rate of use in developing countries may be as high as 95%.[1] In China, 30% to 50% of medications used consists of traditional herbs.[2] In Africa, nearly 80% of individuals use some form of traditional herbal medicine.[3] First-line herbal home medicinal treatments account for 60% in Ghana, Mali, Nigeria, and Zambia. An estimate of use in North America and Europe stated that 50% of the population used herbal medicines at least once in their lifetime as treatment.[4] The number of once in a lifetime-users in Germany and Canada ranged from 70% to 90%. The population of the United States identified as using herbs stands at 158 million adults. This accounts for a significant spending amount of more than $60 billion annually and growing on a global scale.[4,5]

Herbs are used in isolation and as a complement to traditional treatments for physiologic and psychological diseases. Herbs are used for pain management, chronic disease management,[6] and noncommunicable diseases,[7] among others. The combination of herbs and conventional medications can cause life-threatening complications and even lead to death.[8] Despite this fact, the use of herbal medications is world-wide and growing.

HERBAL MEDICATION REGULATIONS

In the United States, herbal medications are regulated by the Food and Drug Administration (FDA) (Dietary Supplements) because they regulate dietary ingredients.[9] Both finished dietary supplement products and dietary ingredients are regulated by this section of the FDA. The Dietary Supplement Health and Education Act of 1994—Public Law 103-417 is federal legislation that defines and regulates dietary supplements. This different set of regulations is different from those used for "conventional" drug products. The FDA works with industry to address concerns about herbal medications that present serious consumer risks. Health care providers should not rely on these FDA notifications alone, and must have some foundational knowledge related to regulations. According to the Dietary Supplement Health and Education Act of 1994:

a. A dietary supplement is a product other than tobacco and includes an herb or other botanicals.
b. Manufacturers and distributors are responsible for evaluating an herbal product for safety and ensuring that it meets Dietary Supplement Health and Education Act of 1994 and FDA regulations.
c. An herbal medication is not required to be approved before public distribution, although FDA petitions may be required for health labeling claims and new ingredients.
d. The FDA monitors consumer-reported problems and issues alerts and safety information through consumer advisories.
e. Warning letters may be issued by the FDA related to adulterated products on the market. Illegal herbal products may be confiscated, and injunctions may be levied against both the manufacturers and distributors.

For many herbal medications, the exact chemical combination that produces a biological effect is unknown and there is no precise chemical fingerprint.[10] As a result of current law and regulations in the United States, there is limited scientific evidence to validate herbal medicinal effects. Unlike conventional medications, herbal medications may be marketed for client use with no clinical tests and minimal proof of efficacy.

It is important for the health care provider to note that to correlate failure of conventional US regulation to a perception of safety and a lack of adverse effects is misleading and untrue.[11] Herbs may produce undesirable effects and adverse reactions as well. These reactions may range from poisoning to death.[12,13] Awareness of real and potential complications must be kept in mind.

HERBS USED IN CARDIOVASCULAR DISEASE: HERB, EFFECT, AND IMPLICATIONS
Garlic

Garlic has traditional dietary and medicinal roles. Traditions related to the use of garlic identified it as a prophylactic and therapeutic intervention for various disease processes. It was used in ancient Chinese and Indian medicine, as well as throughout medieval times.[14] Some of the earliest writings related to the use of garlic was in a collection of Zoroastrian holy writings that possibly date back to the sixth century BC.[15]

Garlic is relatively low in vitamins and minerals; the level of normal consumption only accounts for less than 2% of a daily requirement. The moisture content of garlic is 62% to 68%, which is lower than most fruits and vegetables.[16] Other components of garlic include high levels of fructans, fructose polymers, and common free amino acids.[17] A reportedly unique feature of garlic is its high organosulfur compound content. Ninety-nine percent of these compounds contain the sulfur amino acid cysteine. This percent is 4 times greater than other sulfur-containing fruits and vegetables, such as apricots, onions, and broccoli.[16]

The most abundant sulfur compound in garlic is alliin (S-allycysteine sulfoxide). Cysteine sulfoxides are important parent compounds to several of garlics pharmaceutical effects.[18] Garlic chemically responds differently based on its method of preparation or alteration. Cutting, crushing, or chewing garlic cloves results in the conversion of cysteine sulfoxides to a new compound class, thiosulfinates. Chopping or crushing garlic results in the activation of the alliinase enzyme, which produces allicin from alliin. The principle bioactive compound in aqueous extract or raw garlic is allicin (allyl 2-propenethiosulfinate or diallyl thiosulfinate). Aging garlic extract (garlic stored in 15% to 20% ethanol for >1.5 years) results in a loss of allicin and increased activity in newer compounds with antioxidant properties.[19]

The cardiovascular effects of garlic include lowering of serum lipids, blood pressure, cholesterol, and triglycerides. Garlic is also reported to inhibit platelet aggregation and increase fibrinolytic activity.[20] The suggested mechanism of action for the antihypertensive activity of garlic is due to prostaglandin-like effects. This effect reduces peripheral vascular resistance.[21] The net effect of blood pressure reduction is reportedly 10 to 12 mm Hg for systolic readings[22] and 6 to 8 mm Hg for diastolic readings.[23] Experimentation in rats with induced hypercholesterolemia resulted in a reduction of serum cholesterol, triglycerides and low-density lipoproteins (LDL).[24] In vitro experiments also showed LDL suppression, oxidation and increased high-density lipoproteins. Garlic has been suggested to show a decrease in total serum cholesterol by 17 ± 6 mg/dL and LDL by 9 ± 6 mg/dL. Although there was a significant decrease of LDL, high-density lipoproteins levels did not seem to follow this same improvement level, with a reportedly only slight improvement.[19]

Research has validated a correlation between garlic ingestion and several effects on the cardiovascular system. Several studies suggest that garlic has a direct effect on the cardiovascular system. These studies must be critically reviewed for several reasons, including the (a) study timeframe, because some were of short duration; (b) the type of study, because there were few clinical trials, and (c) the differences in garlic preparation, because these differences can produce various levels of garlic constituents based on preparation and ingestion method.

Owing to the complexity of cardiovascular disease and its prevalence, it is important to consider garlic as a potential complement based on some research to date but only after considering as many client perspectives as possible that may pose a potential risk inclusive of but not limited to age, heredity, condition (eg, pregnancy), and culture. The risk of interactions with current traditional medication treatments must also be considered. The effects of some cardiovascular medications may be potentiated by the ingestion of garlic. One garlic property identified is its reducing effect on platelet function. Ingestion of garlic with aspirin or anticoagulant medications could lead to an increased risk of bleeding.[25] A review of garlic ingestion in all forms is important to investigate.

Ginkgo Biloba

Ginkgo biloba is the oldest living plant species. A tree can live to 1000 years of age. It was identified to exist 150 million years ago during the Mesozoic era.[26] The herb reached its greatest development during the Jurassic and Cretaceous periods. It is referred to as a living fossil.[26,27] Today, gingko biloba is cultivated in many countries including New Zealand, Argentina, North America, Asia, and Europe.[28]

Gingko biloba has been used for centuries in Chinese medicine. Both the gingko leaf and seeds have been used for medicinal purposes. Current research using the gingko plant focuses on using a standardized extract made from dried green leaves. This extract is very concentrated and is purported to have an affect on cardiac conditions.

The main bioactive constituents of gingko biloba are terpene lactones and flavonols. These constituents are reported to be responsible for the herb's therapeutic effects. Terpene lactones are exclusive to ginkgo biloba trees. These lactones comprise diterpenes ginkgolides A, B, C, and J, as well as sequiterpene bilobalide. Terpene lactones are reported to have several cardiovascular effects, which include (a) cardioprotection,[29] (b) endothelial protection,[30] and (c) antiplatelet properties.[31]

Endothelial protective properties are attributed to ginkgolide B. It is identified to have specific platelet activating factor receptive antagonist properties. One study validated that ginkgolide B in combination with CV 3988 inhibited oxidative stress.[32] Intracellular oxidative stress represents free radical and antioxidant imbalance in the body. Acute myocardial infarction causes oxidative stress reactions. These reactions result in the degradation of coronary vessel structures and promote high expressions of the vascular endothelial cell adherence factor in infarcted cardiac muscle tissue. Ginkgo biloba has exhibited a decrease in myocardial infarction size in mice. It was reported to increase levels of serum histamine, and decrease lactate dehydrogenase, creatine kinase, and creatine kinase myocardial band levels.[33]

Ginkgo biloba has been identified to inhibit platelet aggregation induced by agonists, which suggest that it may interfere with a signaling molecule in the platelet activation cascade. It was demonstrated to target a specific kinase that contributes to activation of human platelets to support thrombosis. By specifically targeting this pathway, it produces an antithrombotic effect.[34]

The addition of ginkgo biloba in combination with specific cardiac medications should be carefully considered and all potential effects taken into consideration. There have been some reported risks of ginkgo biloba interacting with antiplatelet and anticoagulant medications and the potential for an idiosyncratic bleeding episode is supported by some evidence.[35] This herb is reported to have some antiplatelet properties of its own, so its combination with traditional medications may enhance this effect, although investigation supports that there may be no increased side effects.[36] The research in this regard, however, is varied. It is imperative for the care provider to compare the risks versus benefits when recommending this herb for cardiac conditions.

Ginseng (Panax Ginseng)

Ginseng has been used for thousands of years in eastern cultures like Korea, China, and Japan. Ginseng is a common name for several species of perennial plants. It belongs to the *Panax* of the Araliaceae family. Its name, *Panax Ginseng*, means *all healing*. Ginseng is still a commonly used herbal medicine not only in oriental countries but worldwide. It is reported to have a range of therapeutic implications. These implications are in addition to its reported pharmacologic application. The most common ginsengs are (a) American ginseng (*P quinquefolium L.*), (b) Chinese ginseng (*P notoginseng*), and Korean red ginseng (*P ginseng Meyer*). The active ginseng constituent, ginsenosides, was identified in 1963.[37] Ginsenosides are the major components and have been identified to contribute to the effects of ginseng. These ginsenoside constituents are thought to have vasorelaxation, antioxidation and anti-inflammatory properties.[38]

Several cardiac effects have been identified from ginseng constituents. Ginsenoside Rb_1 has been identified to have an inhibitory effect on cardiac hypertrophy in the rat model.[39] Ginsenoside Rd has been reported to decrease basilar hypertrophic remodeling in stroke-prone hypertensive rats.[40] Ginsenosides Rg_1, Rg_2, and Rh_1 have been reported to possess both calcium channel blockade and anti–free radical effects.[41] Ginsenoside Rh_1 was reported to affect basic functions of myocardiocytes. This affect resulted in open time reduction, close time increase and open-state probability of calcium channels in myocardiocytes.[41] Studies of ginsenoside Rg_1 reported induced smooth muscle remodeling.[42] Ginsenoside Rg_1 has also reportedly inhibited angiotensin II induced vascular smooth cell proliferation.[43,44] There is a suggestion that ginsenoside Rb_3 from *P ginseng* administration offers protection against isoproterenol-induced myocardial injury and impairment of heart function in the rat model.[43]

Ginseng has been used worldwide to address cardiac and other health problems. There are many studies that report positive outcomes for many ginsenosides. Overall research evidence is conflicting regarding cardiac benefits. Consistency of chemical composition and pharmacologic properties can vary, which can affect safety and effectiveness. It is imperative to validate assertions identified by many research studies. Ginseng clinical trials are increasing in number, but many need clearer and stricter methodologies to demonstrate efficiency of ginseng.[45] The induction properties of cytochrome P450 2C9, a drug-metabolizing enzyme in the body, in ginseng also warrant continued investigation because this mechanism of action is noted to reduce the effect of warfarin.[46]

Green Tea

Tea is popular worldwide as a solo or complementary beverage. Green tea has especially grown in popularity as an intervention to manage cardiovascular disease as information has become more available through technology. Green tea benefits are promoted technologically through access to scholarly and nonscholarly resources. Green tea is the nonoxidized dried leaves of the *Camellia sinensis* plant.[47] The manufacturing of green tea involves polyphenol oxidase inactivation in the fresh leaves.

Green tea contains flavonoids. Flavonoids are naturally occurring polyphenolic compounds. The most abundant flavonoids in green tea are catechins. The major catechins in green tea are (a) epicatechin, (b) epicatechin-3-gallate (ECG), (c) epigallocatechin (EGC), and (d) epigallocatechin-3-gallate (EGCG).[48] Catechins account for 80% to 90% of flavonoids in green tea. The most abundant catechin in green tea is EGCG, which accounts for 48% to 55% of the total catechin amount. The remaining catechin content is EGC at 9% to 12%, ECG at 9% to 12%, and epicatechin at 5% to 7%.[49] Green tea catechin bioavailability is important to consider when looking at its impact on cardiovascular disease. Plasma catechin concentration is increased 2 to 4 hours after consuming green tea.[48] This availability can significantly affect its biological activity within targeted tissues. Catechin bioavailability differs among catechins type with EGCG reportedly less available.[50] A vast majority of major tea catechins are conjugates in plasma. These conjugates retain parent antioxidant abilities and as a result may still exert beneficial results.[51] Catechins have reportedly beneficially affected the multifactorial components of cardiovascular disease, which include vascular tone, inflammation, and proliferation of vascular cells. The cardioprotective effects of green tea include modulation of specific cellular signaling pathways. This pathway modulation leads to reduced inflammation and platelet aggregation, as well as an elevation of vascular activity.[52] Vascular endothelial functioning is also improved through activation of certain endothelial cells.[52]

Green tea catechins have an effect on the lipid profile, which can decrease the potential for hyperlipidemia. Catechins epicatechin, EGC, ECG, and EGCG demonstrate suppression of intracellular lipid accumulation in vitro.[53] Green tea catechins reportedly affect lipid metabolism and prevent atherosclerotic plaque.[54,55] This activity causes a decrease in blood cholesterol levels, which prevents deposition and/or accumulation of cholesterol in the liver and heart in rats.[56] Studies show that the cholesterol-lowering effect of catechins may be due to their ability to interfere with intestinal lipid absorption.[57]

Green tea contains many polyphenolic antioxidants. Polyphenol extraction from green tea is time and temperature dependent.[58] Enzymatic oxidation of green tea catechins occurs by firing or steaming. Preparing green tea with hot water improves its ability to scavenge oxidative radicals. This is identified to likely be due to an ability to better extract polyphenols. Tea polyphenols act as antioxidants in animal studies.[59] Polyphenolic antioxidants in green tea has been reported to demonstrate an inverse relationship between consumption and coronary artery disease. Higher consumption by individuals in Japan resulted in a lower incidence of coronary artery disease.[60]

Green tea popularity is growing among individuals who seek herbal solutions to their cardiovascular conditions. Epidemiologic data from several clinical and experimental studies demonstrate that there may be a positive correlation between consuming green tea and its beneficial effects on cardiovascular health. Although many studies have validated an antioxidant and free radical effect in both animals and humans, there are studies that have demonstrated no effect for tea catechins on plasma antioxidants.[61,62] It is worthy to note that no study reported significant ill physiologic effects from green tea consumption. Side effects were mild and not attributed to the tea intervention. The only caution for green tea use is its reported interaction to antagonize the effect of warfarin because it contains small amounts of vitamin K.[63] Individuals taking warfarin should be cautioned not to consume green tea.

Milk Thistle (Silybum marianum)

Milk thistle (Silybum marianum) was reportedly used as early as 23 AD by Pliny and Elder as a treatment for "carrying off bile."[64] This herb is best known for its effect on the liver. Its use as an antidote for "liver toxins" was first promoted in the middle ages. Milk thistle was later used by physicians Felter and Lloyd for liver "congestion."[65] Native Americans used milk thistle for skin disorders. The herb's preparations have been used for liver dysfunction,[64] alcoholic liver disease and cirrhosis, infectious hepatitis, and drug-induced hepatitis.[66] Milk thistle has been primarily promoted and commonly prescribed as a hepatoprotectant for individuals with cancer. Milk thistle is native to the Mediterranean region (southern Europe, western Asia, and northern Africa). It has become established in parts of Europe, North America, South America, Australia, and New Zealand.[67]

Milk thistle is a mixture of natural substances, but it can have a slightly different composition being plant based.[68] Its ingredients are 70% to 80% flanonolignans (silibinim [silybin], isosilybin, silychristin, isosilychristin, silydianin) and other flanonoids. The remaining 20% to 30% is an undefined flanonoid fraction (Pourova). Silybum marianum's active constituents are 3 isometric flavonolignans: (a) silibinin, (b) silychristin, and (c) silidianin. These 3 constituents are collectively known as silymarin, which is extracted from the seeds of the milk thistle plant.[69]

Silymarin has been identified to have antioxidant, vasorelaxant, and drug-protectant properties. It also is reported to reduce blood pressure, lipids, triglycerides, total cholesterol, and lipoproteins. The antioxidant properties reported for silymarin are achieved by increasing superoxide activity within the erythrocytes and lymphocytes.[70] The flavonolignan silybin A is stated to exhibit vasorelaxant effects ex vivo in rat aorta.[71] Rat experimentation also demonstrated a decrease in serum total lipids, triglycerides, total cholesterol, and lipoproteins.[72] Silymarin decreased doxorubicin–prooxidative activity and ameliorated doxorubicin-induced cardiotoxicity in rats.[73] It had a significant effect in deoxycorticosterone acetate induced hypertension in rats. Silymarin increased antioxidant activity, increased urinary sodium and potassium excretion and subsequently decreased blood pressure in a rat model.[74]

Using physiologic doses of silymarin is reportedly not toxic and it is purportedly accepted as a safe herb.[75,76] Reported adverse effects include headache, epigastric distress, and dermatologic symptoms. The most common symptom is gastrointestinal.[77] Silymarin has also been reportedly safely used in children,[78] during pregnancy[79] and in adults older than 75 years of age.[80]

It is important for the care provider to continue reviewing evolving research related to potentiating or inhibiting effects of silymarin. Overall, it seems to be generally beneficial, but the pharmacologic effects on cardiac disease remain under investigation. There is strong preclinical evidence related to the liver,[64,71] but limited evidence exists related to cardiac effects in humans.

ROLE OF THE ADVANCED PRACTICE NURSE IN HERBAL USE FOR THE CARDIAC CLIENT

The advanced practice nurse must be astutely aware of their client's needs and how to address physiologic and psychological needs in an economic but safe manner. The use of complementary and alternative medicines is increasing as the cost of health care increases exponentially and often exceeds the financial abilities of individuals. The role of the advanced practice nurse is to facilitate health in a manner that promotes wellness and still is attainable and affordable. Advanced practice nurses can increase their knowledge of complementary and alternative medicine by using readily available evidence-based information. This information can be found at several sites (**Table 1**).

Table 1
Evidence-based information sites (alphabetical order)

Resource	Link	Information Available
Cochrane Review	http://www.cochrane.org	Search multiple databases for numerous therapies
National Cancer Institute	https://www.cancer.gov/about-cancer/treatment/cam	Complementary and alternative medicine in cancer
National Cancer Institute – Division of Cancer Treatment & Diagnosis	https://cam.cancer.gov/	Research, health information, international activities
National Center for Complementary and Integrative Health	https://www.nccih.nih.gov/	Health information, research and training
Natural Medicines Database	http://www.naturalmedicinesdatabase.com	Databases (foods, herbs and supplements) Tools (interaction effectiveness adverse effects and pregnancy and lactation checker)

Management of the client taking complementary medicines for cardiovascular conditions involve several considerations. Medication reconciliation must include all herbs as well as over-the-counter medicines. Cultural considerations are important to address because herbal use may be part of the cultural fabric or familial heritage. Interactions are imperative to consider. Medications such as warfarin have a high probability of interactions with several herbs used for cardiovascular conditions. Herbs may not only be used in their tablet form, but as an added complement to foods as a condiment. Herbs must be reviewed when used by specific populations such as older adults, children, and pregnant women. The advanced practice nurse must be aware of herbs and their potential as a medicinal support and the possible hazardous effects. There are several sources for retrieval of such information (**Table 2**).

Table 2
Herb and dietary supplement resources (alphabetical order)

Resource	Link	Information Available
American Botanic Council	https://abc.herbalgram.org/site/SPageServer/?pagename=Homepage	Educational information and herbal library
NeedyMeds Be Med Wise, National Council on Patient Information and Education	https://www.bemedwise.org/health-research-and-reports/health-resources-and-toolkits/	Toolkits and patient information for medication use
Dietary Supplements, FDA	https://www.fda.gov/food/dietary-supplements	Current information on dietary supplements. Information on products and ingredients. Supplemental information for consumers.

(*continued on next page*)

Table 2 (continued)		
Resource	**Link**	**Information Available**
MedlinePlus, National Library of Medicine, NIH	https://medlineplus.gov/ druginformation.html	Drug A to Z information. Browse herbs and supplements to identify effectiveness, usual dose and drug interactions.
National Council for Complementary and Integrative Health	https://www.nccih.nih.gov/ health/herbsataglance	Herbs at a glance – A to Z.
Office of Dietary Supplements, NIH	https://ods.od.nih.gov/ factsheets/ dietarysupplements-HealthProfessional/	Dietary supplement information including what is a dietary supplement, FDA regulations, labeling, health benefits and safety evaluation and resources.
United States Pharmacopeial Convention	https://www.quality-supplements.org/ verified-products/ verified-products-listings	USP listing of verified dietary supplements.

SUMMARY

Herbs have been used for thousands of years. They are used for primary and secondary prevention. Garlic, ginkgo biloba, ginseng, green tea, and milk thistle are only a few of the herbs that may be used by individuals to promote well-being in addition to conventional medications in addressing physiologic conditions. There are other herbs that exist that may have an effect on the cardiovascular system. Although there is research related to specific herbs, there is also much more to learn relative to their effect on the human body and specifically the cardiovascular system. Research is ongoing and the care provider must remain current through deliberate investigation of available studies.

Cardiovascular diseases have multiple debilitating components and often patients are attempting to improve their quality of life through several approaches by taking herbs either alone or in combination with their prescribed medications. The health care provider must have a holistic approach to management of patients with cardiovascular diseases. It is important to approach the patient taking herbal medications with respect and understanding. One must also be knowledgeable regarding not only herbs but the entire patient picture. It is imperative to allow the patient an opportunity to explain their perspective. The care provider must embrace their point of view while displaying compassion and providing factual research-based information to educate the patient on benefits and risks of herbs.

CLINICS CARE POINTS

- Herbs can be used for pain management, chronic disease management and in the treatment of noncommunicable diseases.
- The combination of herbs and conventional medications should be done with caution as they can cause life-threatening complications and even lead to death.

- Medications such as warfarin have a high probability of interactions with several herbs used for cardiovascular conditions.
- The cardiovascular effects of garlic include lowering of serum lipids, blood pressure, cholesterol, and triglycerides. Garlic is also reported to inhibit platelet aggregation and increase fibrinolytic activity resulting in increased bleeding which should be closely monitored when used alone or with other medications.
- Gingko biloba contains terpene lactones which have cardioprotection, endothelial protection and antiplatelet properties. Actions may inhibit platelet aggregation and interfere with the platelet activation cascade. As a result, it may potentially cause idiosyncratic bleeding episodes.
- Gensenosides are thought to have vasorelaxation, antioxidation and anti-inflammatory effects but continued research is needed to validate these properties.
- Green tea catechins which reportedly have multifactorial components of cardiovascular disease which include vascular tone, inflammation, and proliferation of vascular cells. It is reported to antagonize warfarin effects as it contains small amounts of vitamin K. Individuals taking warfarin should be cautioned not to consume green tea.
- Milk thistle is reported to reduce blood pressure, lipids, triglycerides, total cholesterol, and lipoproteins. It contains silmaryn and monitoring for side effects which include headache, epigastric distress and dermatologic symptoms are warranted.

DISCLOSURE

The authors have nothing to disclose.

REFERENCES

1. Tilburt JC, Kaptchuk TJ. Herbal medicine research and global health: an ethical analysis. Bull World Health Organ 2008;86(8):594–9.
2. McQuade JL, Meng Z, Chen Z, et al. Utilization of and attitudes towards traditional Chinese medicine therapies in a Chinese cancer hospital: A survey of patients and physicians. Evid Based Complementary Altern Med 2012;504507. https://doi.org/10.1155/2012/504507.
3. World Health Organization. WHO traditional medicine strategy 2002–2005. Geneva (Switzerland): WHO; 2002.
4. Gunjan M, Naing TW, Saini RS, et al. Marketing trends and future prospects of herbal medicine in the treatment of various disease. World J Pharm 2015;4(9): 132–55.
5. Robinson MM, Zhang X. Traditional medicines: global situation, issues and challenges. *The World Medicines Situation* 2011. Geneve: WHO. Available at: http://digicollection.org/hss/documents/s18063en/s18063en.pdf. Accessed May 1, 2020.
6. Weiss CO. Frailty and chronic diseases in older adults. Clin Geriatr Med 2011;27: 39–52.
7. Benziger CP, Roth GA, Moran AE. The global burden of disease study and the preventable burden of NCD. Glob Heart 2016;11:393–7.
8. Awortwe C, Makiwane M, Reuter H, et al. Critical evaluation of causality assessment of herb-drug interactions in patients. Br J Clin Pharmacol 2018;84(4): 679–93.
9. Dietary Supplements. US Food and Drug Administration. Available at: http://www.fda.gov/food/dietarysupplements/default.htm. Accessed April 12, 2020.

10. Bent S. Herbal medicine in the United States: review of efficacy, safety, and regulation. J Gen Intern Med 2008;23(6):854–9.
11. Ekor M. The growing use of herbal medicines: issues relating to adverse reactions and challenges in monitoring safety. Front Pharmacol 2014;4:177.
12. Cosyns JP, Jadoul M, Squifflet JP, et al. Urothelial lesions in Chinese-herb nephropathy. Am J Kidney Dis 1999;33:1011–7.
13. Ernst E. Toxic heavy metals and undeclared drugs in Asian herbal medicines. Trends Pharmacol Sci 2002;23:136–9.
14. Rivlin RS. Patient with hyperlipidemia who received garlic supplements. Lipid Management. Report from the Lipid Education Council. 1998;3:6-7.
15. Dannesteter J. AVESTA: VENDIDAD: Fargard 20: the origins of medicine. Translated from Sacred Books of the East. American edition. New York: The Christian Literature Company; 1898. Available at: www.avesta.org. Retrieved April 2, 2020.
16. Lawson LD. Garlic: a review of its medicinal effects and indicated active compounds. In: Lawson LD, Bauer R, editors. Phytomedicines of Europe. Chemistry and biological activity. Washington, DC: American Chemical Society; 1998. p. 176–209.
17. Darbyshire B, Henry RJ. Differences in fructan content and synthesis in some *Allium* species. New Phytol 1981;87:249–56.
18. Krest I, Glodek J, Keusgen M. Cysteine sulfoxides and alliinase activity of some Allium species. J Agric Food Chem 2000;48(8):3753–60.
19. Bayan L, Koulivand PH, Gorji A. Garlic: a review of potential therapeutic effects. Avicenna J Phytomed 2014;4(1):1–14.
20. Chan JY, Yuen AC, Chan RY, et al. A review of the cardiovascular benefits and antioxidant properties of allicin. Phytother Res 2013;27:637–46.
21. Rashid A, Khan HH. The mechanism of hypotensive effect of garlic extract. J Pak Med Assoc 1985;35:357–62.
22. Kandziora J. Antihypertensive efficacy and tolerability of garlic preparations [Antihypertensive Wirksamkeit und Vertraglichkeit eines Knoblauch-Praparates (Study 2)]. Arztl Forsch 1988;35:1–8.
23. Auer W, Eiber A, Hertkom E, et al. Hypertension and hyperlipidemia: garlic helps mild cases. Br J Clin Pract Suppl 1990;69:3–6.
24. Kamanna VS, Chandrasekhara N. Effect of garlic on serum lipoproteins cholesterol levels in albino rats rendered hypercholesteremic by feeding cholesterol. Lipids 1982;17:483–8.
25. McEwen BJ. The influence of herbal medicine on platelet function and coagulation: a narrative review. Semin Thromb Hemat 2015;41(3):300–14.
26. Chan P-C, Xia Q, Fu P. Ginkgo biloba leave extract: biological medicinal and toxicological effects. J Environ Sci Health C 2007;25(3):211–44.
27. Shu Z, Shar AH, Shahen M, et al. Pharmacological uses of *Ginkgo biloba* extracts for cardiovascular disease and coronary heart diseases. Int J Pharmacol 2019; 15:1–9.
28. Huh H, Staba EJ. The botany and chemistry of *Ginkgo Biloba* L. J Herbs Spices Med Plants 1991;1(1):91–124.
29. Maerz S, Liu CH, Guo W, et al. Anti-ischaemic effects of bilobalide on neonatal rat cardiomyocytes and the involvement of the platelet-activating factor receptor. Biosci Rep 2011;31(5):439–47.
30. Zhou W, Chai H, Courson A, et al. Ginkgolide A attenuates homocysteine-induced endothelial dysfunction in porcine coronary arteries. J Vasc Surg 2006;44(4):853–62.

31. Cho HJ, Nam KS. Inhibitory effect of ginkgolide B on platelet aggregation in a cAMP- and cGMP-dependent manner by activated MMP-9. J Biochem Mol Biol 2007;40(5):678–83.
32. Zhang S, Chen B, Wu A, et al. Ginkgolide B reduces inflammatory protein expression in oxidized low-density lipoprotein-stimulated human vascular endothelial cells. J Cardiovasc Pharmacol 2011;57(6):721–6.
33. Li Y, Zhang Y, Wen M, et al. Ginkgo biloba extract prevents acute myocardial infarction and suppresses the inflammation- and apoptosis-regulating p38 mitogen-activated protein kinases, nuclear factor-κB and B-cell lymphoma 2 signaling pathways. Mol Med Rep 2017;16(3):3657–63.
34. Shiyong Y, Yijia X, Peng Z, et al. Ginkgo biloba extract inhibits platelet activation via inhibition of Akt. Integr Med Int 2014;1:234–42.
35. Bone KM. Potential interaction of Ginkgo biloba leaf with antiplatelet or anticoagulant drugs: what is the evidence? Mol Nutr Food Res 2008;52(7):764-71.
36. Ryu KH, Han HY, Lee SD, et al. Ginkgo biloba extract enhances antiplatelet and antithrombotic effects of cilostazol without prolongation of bleeding time. Thromb Res 2009;124(3):P328–34.
37. Shibata S, Fujita M, Itokawa H, et al. Studies on the constituents of Japanese and Chinese crude drugs. XI. Panaxadiol, a sapogenin of ginseng roots. Chem Pharm Bull (Tokyo) 1963;11:759–61.
38. Tam DNH, Truong DH, Nguyen TTH, et al. Ginsenoside Rh1: a systematic review of its pharmacological properties. Planta Med 2018;84:139–52.
39. Jiang QS, Huang XN, Dai ZK, et al. Inhibitory effect of ginsenoside Rb_1 on cardiac hypertrophy induced by monocrotaline in rat. J Ethnopharmacol 2007;111:567–72.
40. Cai BX, Li XY, Chen JH, et al. Ginsenoside-Rd a new voltage-independent Ca2+ entry blocker reverses basilar hypertrophic remodeling in stroke-prone renovascular hypertensive rats. Eur J Pharmacol 2009;606:142–9.
41. Jiang Y, Liu W, Wang XM, et al. Calcium channel blockade and anti-free radical actions of panaxatriol saponins in cultured myocardiocytes. Acta Pharmacol Sin 1996;17:138–41.
42. Lee JY, Lim KM, Kim SY, et al. Vascular smooth muscle dysfunction and remodeling induced by ginsenoside Rg_3, a bioactive component of ginseng. Toxicol Sci 2010;117:505–14.
43. Wang T, Yu XF, Qu SC, et al. Ginsenoside Rb_3, inhibits angiotensin II-induced vascular smooth muscle cells proliferation. Basic Clin Pharmacol Toxicol 2010; 107:685–9.
44. Wang T, Yu X, Qu S, et al. Effect of ginsenoside Rb_3 on myocardial injury and heart function impairment induced by isoproterenol in rats. Eur J Pharmacol 2010;636:121–5.
45. He Y, Yang J, Lv Y, et al. A review of ginseng clinical trials registered in the WHO International Clinical Trials Registry platform. Biomed Res Int 2018;7. https://doi.org/10.1155/2018/1843142.
46. Janetzky K, Morreale AP. Probable interaction between warfarin and ginseng. Am J Health Syst Pharm 1997;54(6):692–3.
47. Babu PV, Liu D. Green tea catechins and cardiovascular health: an update. Curr Med Chem 2008;15(18):1840–50.
48. Higdon JV, Frei B. Tea catechins and polyphenols: health effects metabolism and antioxidants functions. Crit Rev Food Sci Nutr 2003;43:89–143.
49. Shahidi F. Antioxidants in food and food antioxidants. Nahrung 2000;44(3):158–63.

50. Van Amelsvoort JM, Van Hof KH, Mathot JN, et al. Plasma concentrations of individual tea catechins after single dose in humans. Xenobiotica 2001;31(12): 891–901.

51. Erdman JW Jr, Balentine D, Arab L, et al. Flavonoids and heart health: proceedings of the ILSI North America flavonoids workshop. May 31–June 1, 2005, Washington, DC. J Nutr 2007;137(3):718S–37S.

52. Shenouda SM, Vita JA. Effects of flavonoid-containing beverages and EGCG on endothelial function. J Am Coll Nutr 2007;26(4):366S–72S.

53. Furuyashiki T, Nagayasu H, Aoki Y, et al. Tea catechin suppresses adipocyte differentiation accompanied by down-regulation of PPARγ2 and C/EBPα in 3T3-L1 cells. Biosci Biotechnol Biochem 2004;68(11):2353–9.

54. Khan SG, Katiyar SK, Agarwal R, et al. Enhancement of antioxidant and phase II enzymes by oral feeding of green tea polyphenols in drinking water to SKH-1 hairless mice: possible role in cancer chemoprevention. Cancer Res 1992;52(14): 4050–2.

55. Miura Y, Chiba T, Tomita I, et al. Tea catechins prevent the development of atherosclerosis in apoprotein E-deficient mice. J Nutr 2001;131(1):27–32.

56. Babu PVA, Sabitha KE, Shyamaladevi CS. Green tea extract impedes dyslipidaemia and development of cardiac dysfunction in streptozotocin-diabetic rats. Clin Exp Pharmacol Physiol 2006;33(12):1184–9.

57. Velayutham P, Babu A, Liu D. Green tea catechins and cardiovascular health: an update. Curr Med Chem 2008;15(8):1840–50.

58. Forester SC, Lambert JD. The role of antioxidant versus pro-oxidant effects of green tea polyphenols in cancer prevention. Mol Nutr Food Res 2011;55(6): 844–54.

59. Yan Z, Zhong Y, Duan Y, et al. Antioxidant mechanism of tea polyphenols and its impact on health benefits. Anim Nutr J 2020. https://doi.org/10.1016/j.aninu.2020. 01.001.

60. Sano J, Inami S, Seimiya K, et al. Effects of green tea intake on the development of coronary artery disease. Circ J 2004;68:665–90.

61. Frei B, Higdon JV. Antioxidant activity of tea polyphenols in vivo: evidence from animal studies. J Nutr 2003;133(10):3275S–84S.

62. Tijburg LB, Mattern T, Folts JD, et al. Tea flavonoids and cardiovascular diseases: a review. Crit Rev Food Sci Nutr 1997;37(8):771–85.

63. Hartley L, Flowers N, Holmes J, et al. Green and black tea for the primary prevention of cardiovascular disease. Cochrane Database Syst Rev 2013;(6):CD009934.

64. Post-White J, Ladas EJ, Kelly KM. Advances in the use of milk thistle (*silybum marianum*). Integr Cancer Ther 2007;6(2):1004–109.

65. Flora K, Hahn M, Rosen H, et al. Milk thistle (*Silybum marianum*) for the therapy of liver disease. Am J Gastroenterol 1998;93(2):139–43.

66. Foster S. Milk thistle: Silybum marianum. Rev edition. Austin (TX): American Botanical Council; 1991. p. 285.

67. Luper S. A review of plants in the treatment of liver disease: part 1. Altern Med Rev 1998;3(6):410–21.

68. Chambers CS, Holečková V, Petrásková L, et al. The silymarin composition...and why does it matter??? Food Res Int 2017;100(3):339–53.

69. Bhattacharya S. Milk thistle (Silybum marianum L. Gaert.) seeds in health. In: Preedy VR, Watson R, Patel VB, editors. Nuts and seeds in health and disease prevention. Academic Press; 2011. p. 759–66.

70. Mayer KE, Mayer RP, Lee SS. Silymarin treatment of viral hepatitis: a systematic review. J Viral Hepat 2005;12:559–67.
71. Pourová J, Applová L, Macáková K, et al. The effect of silymarin flavonolignans and their sulfated conjugates on platelet aggregation and blood vessels ex vivo. Nutrients 2019;11(10):2286.
72. Metwally MA, El-Gellal AM, El-Sawaisi SM. Effects of silymarin on lipid metabolism in rats. World Appl Sci J 2009;6(12):1634–7.
73. Rašković A, Stilinović N, Kolarović J, et al. The protective effects of silymarin against doxorubicin-induced cardiotoxicity and hepatotoxicity in rats. Molecules 2011;16:8601–13.
74. Jadhav GB, Upasani CD. Antihypertensive effect of Silymarin on DOCA salt induced hypertension in unilateral nephrectomized rats. Orient Pharm Exp Med 2011;11:101–6.
75. WenWu J, Lin L, Tsai T. Drug-drug interactions of silymarin on the perspective of pharmacokinetics. J Ethnopharmacol 2009;121:185–93.
76. Toklu HZ, Tunali-Akbay T, Erkanli G, et al. Silymarin, the antioxidant component of silybum marianum, protects against burn-induces oxidative skin injury. Burns 2007;33:908–16.
77. Kren V, Walterova D. Silybin and silymarin – new effects and applications. Biomed Pap 2005;149:29–41.
78. Ladas EJ, Cheng B, Hughes D, et al. Milk thistle (*Silybum marianum*) is associated with reductions in liver function tests (LFTs) in children undergoing therapy for acute lymphoblastic leukemia (ALL). Blood 2006;108(11):1882.
79. Hernandez R, Nazar E. Effects of silymarin in intrahepatic cholestasis of pregnancy. Rev Chil Obstet Ginecol 1982;47(1):22–9.
80. Allain H, Schück S, Lebreton S, et al. Aminotransferase levels and silymarin in de novo tacrine-treated patients with Alzheimer's disease. Dement Geriatr Cogn Disord 1999;10(3):181–5.

Highs, Lows, and Health Hazards of Herbology
A Review of Herbal Medications with Psychotropic Effects

Shannon L. Smith-Stephens, DNP, APRN-BC, SANE[a,b,*]

KEYWORDS

- Herbs • Herbal therapy • Anxiety • Depression • Insomnia
- Complimentary alternative medicine • Complimentary integrative medicine

KEY POINTS

- Identification of the most common herbal therapies with psychotropic effects used by clients.
- Assessment of the pharmacokinetics and unwanted effects of psychotropic drug interactions with herbal therapies.
- Roles of the clinician in empowering clients to safely use herbal medications as a compliment rather than replacement.

INTRODUCTION

Mental health disorders such as depression, anxiety, and insomnia are leading causes of hospitalization and disability for young and middle-aged adults.[1,2] Evidence reveals that approximately one-half of all Americans will be diagnosed with a mental illness at some point in their lifetime.[1] In recent years, complementary and alternative medicine (CAM) or complementary integrative medicine use has been trending upward throughout most socioeconomic classes, cultures, and age categories.[2] Plants and roots have been used as medicinal agents since the beginning of recorded time. The purpose of this article is to review herbal and alternative therapies used to treat anxiety, depression, and insomnia. In particular, indications for use, patient education, and possible interactions with conventional prescribed psychotropic medications will be analyzed.

[a] Morehead State University, Morehead, KY, USA; [b] Shannon L. Smith-Stephens, DNP, APRN-BC, PLLC, Olive Hill, KY, USA
* 6902B Grahn Road, Olive Hill, KY 41164.
E-mail address: s.smithstephens@moreheadstate.edu

Nurs Clin N Am 56 (2021) 137–152
https://doi.org/10.1016/j.cnur.2020.10.010
0029-6465/21/© 2020 Elsevier Inc. All rights reserved.

METHODS

A review of the literature was performed using the electronic databases of PubMed, UpToDate, and The Cochrane Library. A search was conducted using the terms complementary alternative medicine, complementary integrative medicine, herbs, herbal supplements, depression, and anxiety. A further search was conducted on the safety, efficacy, pharmacodynamics, and pharmacokinetics of kava, chamomile, lavender, gingko, ginseng, and St John's wort as well as the psychotropic effects of prescription medications and herbal supplements.

DISCUSSION

The National Center for Complementary and Integrative Health (NCCIH), a division of the National Institutes of Health, defines CAM as "a group of diverse medical and health care systems, practices, and products that are not presently considered to be part of conventional medicine."[4(p1)] Approximately 1 in 4 people in the United States uses CAM, which has led to a multibillion-dollar industry. The federal government developed the NCCIH as a lead agency for scientific research on complementary and integrative health approaches. The NCCIH reports that when a nonmainstream practice is used together with conventional medicine, it is considered complementary. A nonmainstream practice used in place of conventional medicine is considered alternative. The NCCIH defines integrative health care as bringing conventional and complementary approaches together in a coordinated way. Integrative health emphasizes a holistic, patient-focused approach to health care and wellness, including mental, emotional, functional, spiritual, social, and community aspects. The goal of integrative health includes treating the whole person rather than an individual organ system.[3]

Plants have been used for medicinal purposes as long as time has been recorded. All major cultures—Native American, European, South American, Asian, and African cultures—have used botanicals for healing purposes. In the 15th century BCE, Egyptians used saw palmetto for urinary symptoms in men.[4] Hippocrates documented the use of St John's wort for mood ailments in the 5th century BCE.[5] Two-thirds of the first edition of the United States Pharmacopoeia, published in 1820, were botanic substances.[5] Through the first half of the 20th century, medicinal herbs continued to be included in the United States Formulary and the United States Pharmacopoeia. After around 1920, pharmaceutical drugs began replacing herbal therapies in the United States as synthetic drugs were found to have greater pharmacologic effects and greater profitability.[5] More than 120 conventionally used pharmaceuticals are derived from plant species.[5,6]

In 1962, the thalidomide defects prompted congress to pass the Kefauver–Harris Drug Amendment, reassigning herbal medicines to the category of food supplements, which have a lower threshold of required evidence for safety.[7] During the 1990s, the US Food and Drug Administration (FDA) attempted to implement increased regulations for herbal products. In response to increased public interest and use of CAMs, Congress established the National Institutes of Health Office of Alternative Medicine in 1992. Since that time, the National Institutes of Health Office of Alternative Medicine was upgraded to the NCCIH.[8] In 1994, Congress passed the Dietary Supplement Health and Education Act to better define and label dietary supplements.[9] New evidence, an increase in case reports, and publicity of adverse effects and harmful drug–herb interactions have prompted many clinicians, organizations, and consumer groups to call for reform of the Dietary Supplement Health and Education Act.[10] In 2007, the FDA issued new rules requiring Good Manufacturing Practices for dietary supplements, requiring proper labeling, free of adulterants, and manufactured according to specified standards for personnel and equipment. However, there is concern as to whether the Good Manufacturing Practices are being uniformly followed owing to significant flexibility in specifying the quality criteria companies will follow.[11] .

IMPACT OF MENTAL HEALTH DISORDERS

The *Diagnostic and Statistical Manual of Mental Disorders*, fifth edition, defines depression as a common and serious mood disorder characterized by persistent feelings of sadness, hopelessness, and loss of interest in activities once enjoyed, lasting for at least 2 weeks. Diagnostic criteria include experiencing 5 or more symptoms during the same 2-week period and at least 1 of the symptoms should be either depressed mood or loss of interest or pleasure. The symptoms must cause the individual clinically significant distress or impairment in social, occupational, or other important areas of functioning.[12]

The *Diagnostic and Statistical Manual of Mental Disorders*, fifth edition,[12] defines generalized anxiety disorder as excessive anxiety and worry, occurring more days than not for at least 6 months, about a number of events or activities (such as work or school performance). An insomnia disorder is found in individuals who experience recurrent poor sleep quality or quantity that causes distress or impairment in important areas of functioning.[12]

The World Health Organization ranks depression as the single largest contributor to global disability (7.5% of years lived with disability in 2015), whereas anxiety disorders are rated sixth (3.4%).[13] Mental health disorders are very common in the United States, with an estimated 50% of all Americans diagnosed with a mental illness or disorder at some point in their lifetime. Mental illness, such as depression, is the third most common cause of hospitalization in the United States for those aged 18 to 44 years old, and adults living with serious mental illness die on average 25 years earlier than others.[1] The 2016 National Ambulatory Medical Care Survey indicated that 56.8 million visits had a mental, behavioral, or neurodevelopmental disorder as the primary diagnosis.[14]

A nationally representative survey in the United States found that approximately 50% of individuals with self-reported depression had used complementary and alternative therapy within the past year. Individuals treated by a conventional medical clinician, two-thirds reported using both prescription and a type of complementary therapy.[15] Thirty percent to 43% of patients treated in primary care for anxiety use CAM remedies for at least part of their treatment.[16–18] None of the herbal remedies described here have been shown in clinical trials to be clearly effective or ineffective for anxiety symptoms, though trials have suggested that kava and chamomile may reduce anxiety in some people with generalized anxiety disorder.[7]

WHO, WHAT, WHEN, WHERE, AND WHY OF HERBAL THERAPY
What

Complementary therapies are used as adjuncts to conventional care. Complementary therapies are intended to be offered as support rather than replacement, to patients and families with serious medical conditions. Alternative medicine refers to therapies intended to take the place of conventional care. Integrative medicine is a relationship-based care, focusing on the holistic being, making use of all available therapeutic approaches, health care professionals, and disciplines to promote ideal health, wellness and healing. A 2007 nationwide government study, cofunded by the NCCAM, found that $34 billion was spent to seek "natural" means to good health. Cauffield[19] addressed the increase in CAM use among consumers, as well as 46.3% of CAM consumers seeing a specified practitioner. This study also found that only 38.5% of individuals reported CAM use to the health care provider, even though 96% had been seen within the past year. A 2012 national survey identified that more than 30% of adults use health care approaches that are not part of conventional medical care or have origins outside of Western medicine.[3]

Why

Americans reported top reasons for using herbs is similar to other CAMs in that they are frequently used for chronic conditions for which conventional medicine does not offer straightforward answers or cures.[20] Enhancing health and helping with common chronic symptoms or diseases such as memory loss, arthritis, and fatigue are some of the common rationales of CAM users. Herbs are appealing to those who perceive nature as benevolent and healing.[21] Associated with this mistaken perception is that naturally derived products are always safe. Patients may equate "herbal" with terms such as "good," "weak," or "healthy" when evaluating CAM. These perspectives underestimate their potential risks, some of which can be poisonous, potent, or addictive as well as having the potential for serious adverse effects such as hepatotoxicity and anticoagulation. Safety in pregnancy is unknown owing to lack of studies.

Astin[22] found 3 primary hypotheses as to why individuals seek out alternative treatments to Western medicines, which included (1) dissatisfaction in some way with conventional treatment, (2) alternative treatments are seen as offering more personal autonomy and control over health care decisions, and (3) CAM are seen as more compatible with the patients' values, worldview, or beliefs regarding the nature and meaning of health and illness. Astin concluded with little support for the first 2 theories and found that, along with being more educated and reporting poorer health status, the majority of CAM users are doing so owing to finding the alternatives to be more congruent with their own values, beliefs, and philosophic orientations toward health and life (1998). Cauffield also studied the psychosocial factors associated with CAM use with similar findings as well as reporting individual cultural upbringing and ethnicity define the use of CAM. **Fig. 1** identifies Cauffield's findings that patients experiencing chronic health conditions not easily treated with conventional medical therapies tend to be CAM users.

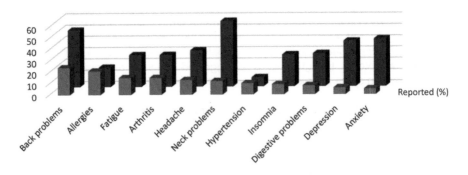

Fig. 1. Adaptation of Cauffield's chronic health conditions and CAM use. (*Adapted from* Cauffield JS. The psychosocial aspects of complementary and alternative medicine. Pharmacotherapy. 2000 Nov;20(11):1289-94. https://doi.org/10.1592/phco.20.17.1289.34898. PMID: 11079276; with permission.)

When and Where

CAM has been used throughout the world, since the beginning of written history. The 2019 World Health Organization Global Report on Traditional and Complementary Medicine indicates that 170 or 88% of all the Member States acknowledged the use of traditional and complementary medicine with 124 or 64% of Member States acknowledging the institution of laws or regulations on herbal medicines.[13]

Who

A 1998 study found that racial or ethnic background as well as sex did not predict the use of CAM; however, education emerged as the single socioeconomic variable that predicted use of CAM. Individuals with higher educational attainment were more likely to use CAM (31% of those with high school or less compared with 50% of those with graduate degrees).[22] This study also found that individuals with declining health status tend to be greater users of CAM. In addition to higher educational levels, CAM users are also found to have higher incomes.[19] As mentioned elsewhere in this article, CAM users tend to have chronic medical conditions such as chronic pain, poor mental health, and cancer, conditions not easily treated by modern medicine. An Australian study found that as many as 79% of the population had used CAM in the previous 12 months. In addition to education, income level, and chronic illness, Thomson and colleagues[23] also found health behaviors, spirituality, openness and prescribing sources to be the strongest predictors of CAM use.

PHARMACOKINETICS AND UNWANTED EFFECTS OF PSYCHOTROPIC DRUG INTERACTION WITH HERBAL THERAPIES
St John's Wort

St John's wort (*Hypericum perforatum*) is a 5-petal yellow flower used medicinally for centuries.[24] The flower is a frequently used herbal therapy in the treatment for depression and anxiety, especially in European countries. In 2002, St John's wort was reported as the sixth most popular naturally used product in the United States, although a decrease was noted in the 2007 NHIS.[16] As with other herbal therapies, mechanism of action is unknown, although numerous compounds have been isolated possessing pharmacologic activity. One such compound, hyperforin, has been shown to modulate neurotransmitter levels, including serotonin, norepinephrine, and dopamine.[25] St John's wort has been primarily used for its antidepressant activity but is also known for anti-inflammatory and wound healing properties.[26] It has been found highly efficacious in vitro against both methicillin-resistant and nonresistant *Staphylococcus aureus*.[27]

St John's wort is frequently used in the treatment of depression. Randomized trials indicate that St John's wort can be efficacious and is generally well-tolerated. However, the American Psychiatric Association recommends clinicians avoid prescribing St John's wort for patients with the initial treatment of major depression owing to the lack of standardization and potency of preparations.[15] Trials have actually found negative results when using St John's wort for anxiety and obsessive-compulsive disorder. St John's wort is more widely used in the management of depression. In a 2008 meta-analysis of randomized clinical trials,[28] Linde and colleagues found hypericum extracts were significantly superior to placebo (95% confidence interval, 1.70–4.01) and, similarly, comparable in efficacy as standard antidepressants for the treatment of mild to moderate depressive disorders. However, results were not observed in similar, older US trials[29] (Hypericurum Depression Study Trial, 2002).

David[30] identified documented adverse effects in patients receiving St John's wort, which may include:

- Photosensitivity
- Nausea
- Fatigue
- Sedation
- Dizziness
- Anxiety
- Dry mouth
- Possible decreased fertility
- Serotonin syndrome

The typical adverse effects when using St John's wort are related to pharmacologic interactions via the cytochrome P450 3A4 pathway.[31] The most common drug reactions include dizziness and confusion, gastrointestinal symptoms, tiredness and sedation, photosensitivity, xerostomia, urinary frequency, anorgasmia, and edema.[32] Drug interactions with a wide variety of pharmaceuticals including anticoagulants, antiretrovirals, antifungals, topical beta-blockers, immunosuppressive agents, narcotics, digoxin, and hormonal contraceptives have been associated with the concomitant use of St John's wort.[7]

A careful review of the medication history is important; clinicians must be mindful regarding importance of education for clients using St John's wort. Patients may self-prescribe St John's wort when psychopharmacologic options have been ineffective or only partially resolve symptoms. The use of St John's wort should be avoided in combination with antidepressants to avert the potential of serotonin syndrome. Documentation of serotonin excess including agitation, hyperthermia, diaphoresis, tachycardia, and neuromuscular disturbances have been reported in older adults taking selective serotonin reuptake inhibitors (SSRIs) and St John's wort simultaneously.[33] Consideration should also be given if switching patients from an SSRI or monoamine oxidase inhibitor (MAOI) to St John's wort. A wash-out period of drug abstinence is recommended; a 3-to 7-day wash-out period is recommended before switching from an SSRI to St John's wort and a 3-week wash-out period before switching from an MAOI to St John's wort.[34] Clinicians should remind patients of the importance of stopping St John's wort at least 5 days before any planned surgical procedure owing to the number of various drug interactions.[35] **Table 1** outlines an adaptation of Bressler's[36] known drug interactions of St John's wort.

CHAMOMILE

Chamomile (*Matricaria recutita*) has been used for centuries for anxiety as well as other conditions. Pittler and Ernst[37] have found evidence of anti-inflammatory, antihyperglycemic, antigenotoxic, and anticancer properties in chamomile using animal research, although none of these effects have been reproduced in human studies. Chamomile's mechanism of action seems to work by binding to gamma aminobutyric acid (GABA) receptors and effecting modulation of monoamine transmission.[38] Clinical trials using chamomile for generalized anxiety disorder have shown mixed results from reducing anxiety on the Hamilton Anxiety (HAM-A) scale compared with placebo to others that have shown no statistical significance between the herbal treatment and placebo.[37]

Topical use of chamomile may cause adverse reactions including hypersensitivity of the skin and mucous membranes. Central nervous system depressants, such as alcohol, should be used with caution with chamomile owing to increased sedative effects. Patients using chamomile should be educated and cautioned regarding increased anticoagulant properties of the herb. Clients requiring anticoagulation

Table 1
Adaptation of Bressler's known drug interactions of St John's Wort

Prescription Drug	Interaction/Effect	Mechanism of Action
Central nervous system A1gents		
Amitriptyline	Blood level decreased 22%. Active metabolite nortriptyline level decreased 41%.	Induction of CYP3A4
Midazolam	Reduced plasma levels	Induction of CYP3A4
Nefazodone	Causes serotonin syndrome; shivering, myoclonus, altered consciousness, central nervous system irritability	Additive effects of inhibition of serotonin reuptake in neuronal cells
Nortriptyline	Decreased plasma concentration 53%	Induction of CYP3A4
Paroxetine	Increased sedative–hypnotic effects (weakness, fatigue, slow movements, incoherent	Combined effects of drugs inhibiting reuptake of neurotransmitters
Quazepam	Decreased plasma concentrations 25% but no clinical effect change	Induction of CYP3A4
Sertraline	Serotonin syndrome	As per paroxetine
Immunologic agents		
Cyclosporine	Decreased blood levels. Caused transplant rejections.	Induction of CYP3A4
Tacrolimus	Decreased plasma concentrations: 6–10 µg/L to 1.6 µg/L. Danger of transplanted organ rejection.	Stimulation of CYP3A4
Antiarrhythmic agents		
Digoxin	Blood levels decreased 25%. Narrow therapeutic index.	Induction of intestinal p-glycoprotein causing digoxin excretion
Antihistamines		
Fexofenadine	Plasma levels and antihistamine activity decreased 35%–45%	Induction of CYP3A4
Cardiovascular agents		
Nifedipine	Decreased plasma concentration 50% and pharmacologic effect	Induction of CYP3A4
Simvastatin	Decreased plasma levels of active metabolite simvastatin hydroxy acid and decreased cholesterol-lowering effect	Induction of CYP3A4
Respiratory agents		
Theophylline	Decreased plasma levels	Stimulation of CYP1A2
Hematologic agents		
Warfarin	Decreased plasma levels and anticoagulant effect	Stimulation of CYP2C9 or inhibition of intestinal absorption is suspected

Adapted from Bressler R. Herb-drug interactions. St. John's wort and prescription medications. Geriatrics. 2005 Jul;60(7):21-3. PMID: 16026178; with permission.

status monitoring with international normalized ratio should be cautioned when chamomile is identified on the medication history.

KAVA-KAVA

Kava-kava or kava (*Piper methysticum*) is used in various cultures for medicinal, religious, and social purposes. The remedy traditionally comes from the root and the principal active ingredients of kava remedies are called kavalactones (15 have been identified, all with psychoactive properties). The mechanism of action for anxiety reduction is not entirely understood, but research suggests involvement of GABA activity and inhibition of norepinephrine and dopamine reuptake.[38–40]

A meta-analysis of 7 randomized trials of 380 participants with elevated anxiety symptoms found that kava extract reduced anxiety as measured by the HAM-A scale compared with participants receiving placebo (weighted mean difference; 3.9; 95% confidence interval, 0.1–7.7).[37] A Cochrane review of 11 randomized controlled trials with rigorous methodology, using 60 mg to 280 mg of kavalactones, revealed statistically significant anxiolytic activity of kava compared with placebo in all but 1 trial.[37] In one 3-arm randomized controlled trial, kava was demonstrated to be equally as efficacious as buspirone and opipramol when treating generalized anxiety disorder in the outpatient setting.[41] Sarris and colleagues[39] did a follow-up double-blind, randomized study, this time with a placebo-controlled study group, finding standardized kava in doses of 120 mg to 250 mg of kavalactones is a moderately effective short-term treatment for generalized anxiety disorder.

Side effects of kava include headaches, sedation, and sleepiness. The literature provides evidence indicating that kava can potentially enhance performance on cognitive tasks, such as working memory and visual processing; however, motor skills, such as reaction time when driving, can be significantly impaired.[38] Heavy, frequent kava users have shown dermatologic findings such as dry, scaling skin as well as increased hepatic transaminase levels. Specific cultures, such as Pacific Island societies, tend to use higher doses in powered form (50–200 g/d), where the medicinal use of kava in tablet form has a lower recommended dose, averaging 6 g/d.[42] There have been numerous reports of severe hepatotoxicity and liver failure, in both Europe and the United States, occurring within a few weeks to up to 2 years (average, 4.5 months) after ingestion of kava.[43] In 2002, the US FDA advised that kava should be used with caution in patients with preexisting liver disease or at risk for liver disease. Pauls and Senior[44] reiterated this advice in a 2012 FDA training course.

Although no specific pharmacokinetic interactions between kava and prescription medications have been documented, kava does have an inhibitory effect on the CYP450 system. This action does potentiate the possibility of drug toxicities when kava is combined with prescription medications with a narrow therapeutic window. Common psychotropic agents metabolized via the CYP450 pathway include diazepam, caffeine, amitriptyline, imipramine, propranolol, fluoxetine, haloperidol, morphine, and beta-blockers.[45] Like benzodiazepines, kava has a rapid onset of action and may be more applicable for intermittent use when acute anxiolytics are necessary. Owing to the similarities of kava and benzodiazepines, monitoring for addiction or abuse is recommended, although medicinal doses have not revealed addiction in the literature.[38] Careful monitoring of transaminase levels and hepatic functioning, alcohol history and education to avoid alcohol, as well as frequent medication list review for concomitant use of medications metabolized by the CYP450 pathway, are necessary interventions for the clinician providing care to the patient using kava as a complementary integrative medicine therapy.

LAVENDER

More than 200 species of *Lavendula* are known, but *L angustifolia* is the most popular species used in lavender oil. Lavender is most well-known for its use as a sedative to relieve insomnia as well as anxiety, although it may also be beneficial in the healing of superficial wounds. The flowering heads of the plant are used for medicinal purposes. Key active components are linalyl acetate and linalool, which occur in varying amounts depending on the species.[46] Lin and colleagues[47] described the mechanism of action as acting directing on the olfactory nerve, producing a sedative effect when inhaled. Other findings reveal the mechanism of action as possibly via the modulation of GABA.[48]

Several studies have provided evidence for the use of lavender. A double-blind, randomized study of the lavender oil preparation, silexan, was compared with lorazepam for generalized anxiety disorder found that silexan was as effective as lorazepam in adults with generalized anxiety disorder as evidenced by decreased HAM-A sub-scores. The results suggest that silexan effectively ameliorates generalized anxiety comparable to a common benzodiazepine (lorazepam). The mean of the HAM-A total score decreased clearly and to a similar extent in both groups (by 11.3 ± 6.7 points [45%] in the silexan group and by 11.6 ± 6.6 points [46%] in the lorazepam group, from 25 ± 4 points at baseline in both groups).[49] Another randomized controlled trial supports the use of lavender and sleep hygiene as safe, accessible, and effective interventions for self-reported sleep issues in college students. Lavender and sleep hygiene together, and sleep hygiene alone to a lesser degree, improved sleep quality for college students with self-reported sleep issues, with an effect remaining at follow-up.[50] These results demonstrate that silexan is as effective as lorazepam in adults with generalized anxiety disorder. The safety of silexan was also demonstrated. Because lavender oil showed no sedative effects in the aforementioned study and has no potential for drug abuse, silexan seems to be an effective and well-tolerated alternative to benzodiazepines for amelioration of generalized anxiety. A systematic review concluded that aromatherapy with lavender oil seemed to be safe and efficacious in decreasing anxiety symptoms in patients with cancer and in patients with dementia receiving palliative care.[49] Skidmore-Roth[51] identified documented adverse effects in patients receiving *Lavendula*, which may include:

- Headache
- Drowsiness
- Dizziness
- Euphoria
- Nausea and vomiting
- Increased appetite
- Constipation
- Contact dermatitis

Clients may self-prescribe lavender, such as lavender aromatherapy, causing the need for clinicians to be aware of possible drug interactions. Central nervous system depressants such as alcohol, antihistamines, opioids, and sedative hypnotics should be avoided owing to the possibility of increased sedation with concurrent use. Lavender may decrease action of hydroxy-3-methyl-glutaryl-coenzyme A reductase inhibitors, as well as decrease absorption of iron.[51]

GINSENG

Asian ginseng (*Panax ginseng*) is a root native to the Far East; American ginseng (*Panax quinquefolius*), another type of ginseng, both of which have been used for thousands of years for medicinal purposes. Chemical components called ginsenosides (or panaxosides) are thought to contribute to the herb's claimed health-related prosperities.[3] Lee and Rhee[52] discussed findings that ginseng has been found to decrease stress and improve coping abilities with anxiety, as well as aiding with memory and improved cognition, concentration, and overall well-being.

Ginseng's mechanism of action has been recognized as a powerful antioxidant that works by reducing the inflammatory response. Ginsenosides have been identified as the active components with health-related properties that act as a platelet activating factor inhabitants as well as having anticancer, antidepressant, and anticonvulsant properties Lee and Rhee.[52]

The literature does not provide any conclusive evidence supporting the health benefits of ginseng. Past studies have been flawed owing to poor methodology. Adverse reactions of ginseng include anxiety, insomnia, chest pain, hypertension, prolonged QT interval, edema, nausea and vomiting, diarrhea, and rash.[51] The National Center for Complementary and Integrative Health[3] has documented numerous drug interactions, which may include:

- Anticoagulants and antiplatelets
- Anticonvulsants
- Antidiabetics including insulin
- Immunosuppressants
- MAOIs
- SSRIs
- Stimulants such as caffeine

GINGKO BILOBA

Saper[53] stated that the ginkgo tree is the world's oldest living tree species, as well as one of the most studied and commonly used herbal remedies in the world. Gingko has been used medicinally for more than 1000 years and was originally used by traditional Chinese clinicians for a variety of conditions, including digestive disorders and asthma. More recently, the ginkgo leaf extract has been used for a number of vascular problems, the treatment of memory loss, dementia, depression, anxiety, and macular degeneration, as well as its antioxidant properties.

Saper[53] discussed 2 main groups of active constituents responsible for Ginkgo biloba's purported medicinal effects: terpene lactones and ginkgo flavone glycosides. Sarris and colleagues[38] identified Gingko biloba's psychopharmacologic mechanism of actions through modulation of cholinergic and monoamine pathways as well as GABA-nergic effects.

A 4-week randomized controlled trial using varying doses of Gingko extract Egb 761 versus placebo revealed a dose-dependent significant decrease of anxiety over placebo of 2.2 and 6.5 points HAM-A for the 480 mg and 240 mg doses of Egb 761, respectively.[38] Saper[53] discussed a study of 40 older adult patients with depression comparing treatment with Gingko biloba extract and placebo. The average total score on the Hamilton Depression Scale decreased significantly after 4 weeks in those treated with Gingko biloba extract compared with placebo.

Skidmore-Roth[51] identified documented adverse effects in patients receiving Gingko biloba, which may include:

- Headache
- Anxiety
- Restlessness

Table 2
Significant patient and provider education on CAM and herbal therapies

	Important Patient Education	Important Provider Education
St John's wort	Photosensitivity: use sunscreen; avoid alcohol and alcohol containing products; caution owing to numerous drug interactions	Wash-out periods of 7–21 d when switching from SSRIs or MAOIs; numerous drug interactions; stop 14–21 d before surgery; significant effect on drugs with peak and trough concentrations
Chamomile	Anticoagulant properties and need to avoid with prescribed anticoagulant medications	Cautious monitoring of international normalized ratio with anticoagulants
Kava-kava	Avoid alcohol and alcohol containing products; caution to caution with heavy machinery owing to drowsiness; possibly habit-forming	Monitor hepatic functioning especially with known liver disease; careful alcohol history; avoid >3 mo owing to possibility of dependence
Lavender	Avoid alcohol and central nervous system depressants owing to increased sedation	May decrease action of 3-hydroxy-3-methyl-glutaryl-coenzyme A reductase inhibitors and iron absorption
Ginseng	Caution owing to numerous drug interactions	Assess for concurrent use of stimulants, anticoagulants, SSRIs, MAOIs, antidiabetics
Gingko biloba	Caution owing to numerous drug interactions	Assess for concurrent use of anticoagulants, SSRIs, MAOIs, platelet inhibitors

- Potential bleeding
- Nausea and vomiting
- Anorexia
- Diarrhea
- Flatulence
- Rash

Potential drug interactions include anticoagulants and nonsteroidal anti-inflammatory drugs, which may lead to decreased platelet activity. Other potential drug interactions include anticonvulsants, Buspirone, some SSRIs, MAOIs, CYP450 substrates, and trazodone. Gingko has been found to decrease the effects of anticonvulsant medications while increasing the effects of MAOIs. Gingko in conjunction with buspirone and fluoxetine may cause hypomania and has been found to cause coma when used simultaneously with trazodone.[51]

EMPOWERING CLIENTS

A review of the literature provides consistent findings that clients do not divulge CAM use to their health care providers. Cauffield[19] investigated why patients do not tell their health care providers they are using CAM. Surveys found that providers who recommended CAM therapies were more likely to be told about use from their patients, but only 25.8% reported using herbal medicine therapies, thus increasing their risk for adverse reactions. Surveys have reported the following rationales as to why patients do not tell their health care providers about CAM use[19,54]:

- Limitations and narrow-mindedness on the part of the health care provider
- Disinterest from the provider
- Lack of questions from provider
- Anticipated negative provider response, unwillingness and inability to help
- Irrelevance of disclosure

Health care practitioners must be able to discern their own values and biases from objective, evidence-based data while also ensuring that clinical practice can retain some artistic elements.[19] As discussed elsewhere in this article, negative pathologic findings of liver dysfunction are a major adverse reaction concern. The United States Drug-Induced Liver Injury Network found approximately 15% to 20% of cases of drug-induced liver injury can be attributed to herbal and dietary supplements.[55] Health care practitioners must remember to investigate the possible use of CAM in a nonjudgmental manner, educating on the possible adverse drug effects and drug–herb interactions that may occur.

Clinicians have an important role in educating patients about herbal remedies. A critical element includes warnings that safety and efficacy of these products for anxiety symptoms and disorders are still unproven, and provide guidance when weighing the risks and benefits of using CAM adjunctively. Patients should be discouraged from abandoning evidence-based psychotherapies and medications for the treatment of mental health disorders. **Table 2** identifies important patient education points regarding the use of herbal remedies.

SUMMARY

Client's use of CAM has created the need for health care practitioners to be informed of current practices and literature related to its use. Though evidence has grown for the use of CAM in the last decade, there continues to be a need for double-blind, randomized controlled trials supporting the use of herbal supplements. The provider must consider the importance of reviewing the medical history and current medication regimen, which should always include over-the-counter medications as well as herbs and supplements. A patient's medical history should include what remedies and supplements they are taking, particularly those known to interact with other drugs or cause adverse effects. CAM should be included in visit histories and discussed in an objective, nonjudgmental manner to encourage patient disclosure.

DISCLOSURE

The author has nothing to disclose.

REFERENCES

1. CDC. National center for health statistics, . Mental health data for the U. S. HYPERLINK ". 2018. Available at: https://www.cdc.gov/nchs/fastats/mental-health. htm. Accessed May 3, 2017.
2. Clarke TC, Black LI, Stussman BJ, et al. Trends in the use of complementary health approaches among adults: United States, 2002-2012. Natl Health Stat Report 2015;10(79):1–16.
3. National Center for Complementary and Integrative Health (2016). Strategic plan: exploring the science of complementary and integrative health. U. S. Department of health and human services. 2018. NCCIH, 4, p1. Available at: https://nccih.nih. gov/sites/nccams.nih.gov/files/NCCIH_2016_Strategic_Plan.pdf.
4. Wilt TJ, Ishani A, Stark G, et al. Saw palmetto extracts for treatment of benign prostatic hyperplasia: a systematic review. JAMA 1998;280(18):1604.
5. Blumenthal M. The ABC clinical guide to herbs. NY: American Botanical Council/ Thieme; 2003.
6. Choffnes D. Nature's pharmacopeia: a world of medicinal plants. NY: Columbia University Press; 2016.
7. Saper R. Clinical use of St. John's wort. UpToDate. 2019. Available at: https:// www-uptodate-com.msu.idm.oclc.org/contents/clinical-use-of-st-johns-wort? search=complimentary%20and%20alternative%20medicine&topicRef=14624&-source=see_link. Accessed January 27, 2020.
8. NIH. National Center for Complimentary and Integrative Health. Asian ginseng. 2016. Available at: https://www.nccih.nih.gov/health/asian-ginseng. Accessed January 27, 2020.
9. Swann JP. The history of efforts to regulate dietary supplements in the USA. Drug Test Anal 2015;8(3–4):271.
10. Marcus DM. Botanical medicines-the need for new regulations. N Engl J Med 2002;347(25):2073.
11. Saper2 R. Overview of herbal medications and dietary supplements. UpToDate. 2019. Available at: https://www-uptodate-com.msu.idm.oclc.org/contents/over-view-of-herbal-medicine-and-dietary   supplements?search=botanical%20medi-cines%20marcus&source=search_result&selectedTitle=1~37&usage_type="' default&display_rank=1.
12. American Psychiatric Association. Diagnostic and statistical manual of mental disorders. 5th edition. Washington, DC: CBS; 2013.
13. WHO Global report on traditional and complimentary medicine. Global report on traditional and complementary medicine 2019. License: CC BY-NY-SA 3.0 IGO. Geneva (Switzerland): World Health Organization; 2019. Available at: https://

www.who.int/traditional-complementary-integrative-medicine/WhoGlobalRepor-tOnTraditionalAndComplementaryMedicine2019.pdf?ua=1.

14. NIH. National Center for Complimentary and Integrative Health. Statistics from the national health interview survey 2017. Available at: https://www.nccih.nih.gov/health/statistics-from-the-national-health-interview-survey. Accessed February 13, 2020.

15. Gitlin M. Unipolar depression in adults and initial treatment: investigational and nonstandard approaches. 2020. Available at: https://www-uptodate-com.msu.idm.oclc.org/contents/unipolar-depression-in-adults-and-initial-treatment-investi-gational-and-nonstandard-approaches?search=herbal%20supplements%20and%20depression%20in%20primary%20care&source=search_result&selec-tedTitle=3~150&usage_type=default&display_rank=3. Accessed January 27, 2020.

16. Barnes PM, Bloom B, Nahin R. Complementary and alternative medicine use among adults and children: United States, 2007. Natl Health Stat Report 2008;(12):1–23.

17. Barnes PM, Powell-Griner E, McFann K, et al. Complementary and alternative medicine use among adults: United States, 2002. Adv Data 2004;27(343):1–19.

18. Bystritsky A, Hovav S, Sherbourne C, et al. Use of complementary and alternative medicine in a large sample of anxiety patients. Psychosomatics 2012;53(3):266–72.

19. Cauffield JS. The psychosocial aspects of complementary and alternative medicine. Pharmacotherapy 2000;20(11):1289–94.

20. Kaufman DW, Kelly JP, Rosenberg L, et al. Recent patterns of medication use in the ambulatory adult population of the United States: the Slone survey. JAMA 2002;287(3):337.

21. Kaptchuk TJ, Eisenberg DM. The persuasive appeal of alternative medicine. Ann Intern Med 1998;129(12):1061.

22. Astin JA. Why patients use alternative medicine: results of a national study. JAMA 1998;279(19):1548–53.

23. Thomson P, Jones J, Browne M, et al. Psychosocial factors that predict why people use complementary and alternative medicine and continue with its use: a population based study. Complement Ther Clin Pract 2014;20:302–10.

24. Hobbs C. St. john's wort-ancient herbal protector. Pharm Hist 1990;32(4):166.

25. Yoshitake T, Iizuka R, Yoshitake S, et al. Hypericum perforatum L (St John's wort) preferentially increases extracellular dopamine levels in the rat prefrontal cortex. Br J Pharmacol 2004;142(3):414–8. https://doi.org/10.1038/sj.bjp.0705822.

26. DerMarderosian A, Liberti L, Beutler J, et al. Review of natural products. St Louis (MO): Facts and comparisons. Wolters Kluwer Health; 2014.

27. Gerstel J, Turner T, Ruiz G, et al. Identification of botanicals with potential therapeutic use against methicillin-resistant Staphylococcus aureus (MRSA) infections. Phytother Res 2010;32(12):2577.

28. Linde K, Berner L, Kriston L. St. John's wort for major depression (review). Cochrane Database Syst Rev 2008;4:CD000448.

29. Fava M, Alpert J, Nierenberg A, et al. A double-blind, randomized trial of St. John's wort, fluoxetine, and placebo in major depressive disorder. J Clin Psychopharmacol 2005;25(5):441–7.

30. David ST. Drug interactions facts: herbal supplements and food. Facts and Comparisons. St. Louis (MO): A. Walters Kluwer Company; 2004. Available at: www.factsandcomparisons.com.

31. Roby CA, Anderson GD, Kantor E, et al. St. John's wort: effect on CYP3A4 activity. Clin Pharmacol Ther 2000;67:451–7.

32. Knuppel L, Linde K. Adverse effects of St. John's wort: a systematic review. J Clin Psychiatry 2004;65(11):1470–9.

33. Wong AH, Smith M, Boon HS. Herbal remedies in psychiatric practice. Arch Gen Psychiatry 1998;55(11):1033.

34. Hirsch M, Birnbaum R. Selective serotonin reuptake inhibitors: pharmacology, administration, and side effects. 2019. Available at: https://www.uptodate.com/contents/selective-serotonin-reuptake-inhibitors-pharmacology-administration-and-side-effects. Accessed February 3, 2020.

35. Wong A, Townley SA. Herbal medicines and anaesthesia. jContin Edu Anesth Crit Care Pain 2011;11(1):14–7.

36. Bressler R. Herb-drug interactions. St. John's wort and prescription medications. Geriatrics 2005;60(7):21–3.

37. Pittler MH, Ernst E. Kava extract for treating anxiety. Cochrane database Syst Rev 2003;(1):CD003383.

38. Sarris J, LaPorte E, Schweitzer I. Kava: a comprehensive review of efficacy, safety, and psychopharmacology. Aust N Z J Psychiatry 2011;45(1):27.

39. Sarris J, McIntyre E, Camfield DA. Plant-based medicines for anxiety disorders, part 1: a review of preclinical studies. CNS Drugs 2013;27(3):207–19.

40. Teschke R, Schwarzenboeck A, Hennermann KH. Kava hepatoxicity: a clinical survey and critical analysis of 26 suspected cases. Eur J Gastroenterol Hepatol 2008;20(12):1182.

41. Boerner RJ, Sommer H, Berger W, et al. Kava-kava extract LI 150 is as effective as opipramol and buspirone in generalized anxiety disorder-an 8-week randomized, double-blind multi-centre clinical trial in 129 out-patients. Phytomedicine 2003;10(4):38–49.

42. Clough A. Enough! Or too much. What is "excessive" kava use in Arnhem Land? Drug Alcohol Rev 2003;22:43–51.

43. CDC. Food and Drug Administration consumer advisory: kava-containing dietary supplements may be associated with severe liver injury. MMWR Morb Mortal Wkly Rep 2002;51(47):1065.

44. Pauls L, Senior J. Drug-induced liver injury. Clinical investigator training course. College Park (MD), November 15, 2012.

45. Singh YN. Potential for interaction of kava and St. John's wort with drugs. J Ethnopharmacol 2005;100(1–2):108–13.

46. Fismer K, Pilkington K. Lavender and sleep: a systematic review of the evidence. Eur J Integr Med 2012;e436–47. Available at: www.sciencedirect.com.

47. Lin PW, Chan W, Ng BF, et al. Efficacy of aromatherapy (Lavendula angustifolia) as an intervention for agitated behaviours in Chinese older persons with dementia: a cross-over randomized trial. Int J Geriatr Psychiatry 2007;22:405–10.

48. Yamada K, Yoshihiro M, Sashida Y. Effects of inhaling the vapor of Lavandula Burnatii super-derived essential and linalool on plasma adrenocorticotropic hormone (ACTH), catecholamine and gonadotropin levels in experimental menopausal female rats. Biol Pharm Bull 2005;28(2):378–9.

49. Bystritsky A. (2020). Complementary and alternative treatments for anxiety symptoms and disorders: herbs and medications. UpToDate. Available at: https://www-uptodate-com.msu.idm.oclc.org/contents/complementary-and- alternative-treatments-for-anxiety-symptoms-and-disorders-herbs-andmedications?search=complementary%20and%20alternative%20symptoms%20for%anxiety&

source=search_result&selectedTitle=1~150&usage_type=default&display_ rank=1. Accessed February 3, 2020.

50. Lillehei A, Halcon L, Kay S, et al. Effect of inhaled lavender and sleep hygiene on self-reported sleep issues: a randomized control trial. J Altern Complement Med 2015;21(7):430–8.

51. Skidmore-Roth L. Mosby's handbook of herbs & natural supplements. 4th edition. St Louis (MO): Mosby Elsevier; 2010.

52. Lee & Rhee. Effects of ginseng on stress-related depression, anxiety, and the HPA axis. J Ginseng Res 2017;41:589–94.

53. Saper R. Clinical use of gingko biloba. UpToDate. 2018. Available at: https:// www-uptodate-com.msu.idm.oclc.org/contents/clinical-use-of-ginkgo-biloba? search=ginkgo%20biloba&source=search_result&selectedTitle=1~49&us- age_type=default&display_rank=1. Accessed February 3, 2020.

54. Jou J, Johnson P. Nondisclosure of complementary and alternative medicine use to primary care physicians. Findings from the 2012 national health interview sur- vey. JAMA Intern Med 2016;176(4):545–6.

55. Larson A. Hepatotoxicity due to herbal supplements. UpToDate. 2020. Available at: https://www-uptodate-com.msu.idm.oclc.org/contents/hepatotoxicity-due-to- herbal-medications-and-dietarysupplements?search=hepatotoxicity%20due% 20to%20herbal%20supplments&source=search_result&selectedTitle=1~150& usage_type=default&display_rank=1.

Healthy Uses for Garlic

Danielle White, MSN, RN

KEYWORDS

- Garlic • Herbal medicine • Anti-inflammatory • Antioxidant • Hypolipidemia

KEY POINTS

- Garlic has been used for health since the time before Christ.
- Early uses of garlic had to do with its antibacterial qualities.
- Fresh garlic has the most health benefits.
- Garlic has been shown to decrease serum cholesterol and triglycerides.

INTRODUCTION AND HISTORY

According to the online Merriam-Webster dictionary, garlic is "a European allium (*Allium sativum*) widely cultivated for its pungent compound bulbs much used in cookery *broadly*: ALLIUM".[1] It also is defined as "a plant of the onion family that has a strong taste and smell and is used in cooking to add flavor".[2] Currently most of the world's garlic grows in Central Asia, followed by India.

A Short History of Garlic

Garlic originated in Central Asia, specifically from Western China, spreading to Japan and Korea.[3,4] From 2600 BCE to 2100 2600 BCE, the Sumerians used garlic for its health qualities.

In 2700 BCE, in ancient China, garlic was used for its stimulating and heating effects. It was the yang, the positive image (in the yin and yang concept). Garlic was recommended to those who suffered depression.

In ancient Indian medicine, garlic was used as a tonic to cure a multitude of diseases (lack of appetite, common weakness, cough, skin disease, rheumatism, and hemorrhoids). In these cases, spells, ritual, and prayers accompanied the healing.

The ancient Israelis made use of garlic as a starvation stimulator, blood pressure enhancer, body heater, parasite killer, and so forth. The Talmud, the book of Judaism, prescribes a meal with garlic every Friday.

The ancient Greeks also valued garlic, although those who had eaten garlic were forbidden entry into the temples. Early Greek army leaders fed their army with garlic before major battles. It is an interesting fact that although nowadays some athletes

School of Nursing, Austin Peay State University, McCord, Room 218, P.O. Box 4658, Clarksville, TN 37044, USA
E-mail address: whited@apsu.edu

Nurs Clin N Am 56 (2021) 153–156
https://doi.org/10.1016/j.cnur.2020.12.001
0029-6465/21/© 2020 Elsevier Inc. All rights reserved.

take a wide spectrum of dangerous tranquilizers, Greek Olympic athletes eat garlic to ensure a good score.

In his works, Hippocrates (459–370 BCE) mentioned garlic as a remedy against intestinal parasites and as a diuretic. Dioscorides (40–90 CE) recommended garlic as a remedy for colic relief, as an anthelmintic, and for regulating the menstruation cycle and against seasickness. He and the Romans recommended garlic as a remedy against snakebite (for that purpose they drank a mixture of garlic and wine) and against mad dog's bite (for that purpose, they applied garlic on the wound directly). Hence, the Greeks called garlic a snake-grass.

In the seventh century CE, the Slavic people used garlic against lice, spider bite, snakebite, and ulcers and crusts.

Garlic was brought into Great Britain in 1548, from the coasts of the Mediterranean Sea, where it was present in abundance. Wild garlic was growing and was cultivated in church courtyards in England for centuries. Teas and tinctures were made and added to honey to beat many gastric infections and to fight cold, fever, and diarrhea, thereby prolonging the lives of many sick people.

In 1858, Louis Pasteur wrote that garlic killed bacteria. As he maintained, it was effective even against some bacteria resistant to other factors. He also noted that garlic killed *Helicobacter pylori*.

The antiseptic properties of garlic were confirmed in the minimizing the incidence of cholera (in 1913), typhoid fever, and diphtheria (in 1918) in Beirut, Lebanon. French phytotherapist Lekrek used garlic as a preventive remedy with success during the great pandemic of influenza, the so-called "Spanish fever", in 1918. During the epidemic of influenza in America during 1917 and 1918, people wore a necklace of garlic when going out in public.

Garlic also is known as Russian penicillin because Russian physicians have used it for a long time for treatment of respiratory tract diseases, and, along with other compounds, it was used as an inhalator remedy for children.

How to Use

Garlic cloves can be eaten raw, cooked, powdered, or pressed into tablets. The principal active compound in garlic is allicin. The most health benefits come from fresh garlic. Once garlic is chopped or crushed, the enzyme is activated but is present only for a short time. Leaving the crushed garlic sit for 10 minutes may prevent the loss of some of the healing properties.[1,5] Garlic supplements often do not include allicin.

Health benefits of garlic include the prevention and treatment of cardiovascular disease, antioxidant effects, antimicrobial effects, and reduction of cancer risks.

HEALTH BENEFITS OF GARLIC
Cardiovascular Disease

Garlic has a significant effect on "lowing blood pressure, prevention of atherosclerosis, reduction of serum cholesterol and triglyceride inhibition of platelet aggregation and increasing fibrinolytic activity".[6] In the arteries, aged garlic extract can slow the progression of arterial plaque by 80%.[7] Additionally, garlic can reduce total cholesterol and low-density lipoprotein (LDL) cholesterol and decrease systolic blood pressure and diastolic blood pressure.

Antiobesity and Hypolipidemic Effects

In 1 study, rats were given a combination of garlic oil and onion oil while being encouraged to gain weight through feeding a high fat diet.[7] Results demonstrated that the body weight gain and lipid levels in the rats fed the oils were decreased significantly. When applied to human health, garlic and onions are readily available and can provide similar effects of antiobesity and hypolipidemia.

Although not all research agrees, the most reliable evidence shows that taking garlic may reduce total cholesterol and LDL, or bad, cholesterol in people with high cholesterol levels. Garlic appears to work best if taken daily for more than 8 weeks, but any benefit is probably small. And taking garlic does not help increase high-density lipoprotein, or good, cholesterol or lower levels of other blood fats, called triglycerides.[8]

Antimicrobial Effects

Garlic incorporated daily into the diet provides many positive effects. Again, the allicin created by cut garlic attacks and kills whatever it is threatened by. It is effective for various bacteria, viruses, and fungi, including staphylococcus, streptococcus, klebsiella, bacillus, and H pylori, to name a few.[2,3,9] According to a study of the American Medical Association, combining traditional antibiotic therapy with natural options may increase the effects of therapy. Many garlic supplements do not contain allicin, so incorporating raw garlic into a diet daily may be therapeutic. Additionally, there is a process to freeze-dry garlic to maintain potency.

One study looked at the antibacterial and antiviral effects of garlic related to the common cold. The active ingredients in garlic are supposed to boost the immune system, thus reducing the common cold. Although there were fewer reports of the common cold in those who took garlic with active allium, the results demonstrated insufficient evidence to confirm the effects on the common cold.[10] More studies are needed to validate this finding.

Anti-inflammatory Effects

The oil and extracts of garlic have anti-inflammatory, antibacterial, fibrinolytic, and wound-healing properties that may make it a substitute for classic antibiotics and antiseptics.

Administering garlic oil to female rats reduced postoperative inflammation. The sulfur-containing compounds in garlic extracts accelerate the formation of new tissue and activated blood supply to open wounds.[11]

Diabetes

One study confirms that additional garlic contributes to reduce premeal blood sugar levels in type 2 diabetes mellitus if taken for at least 3 months as part of supplementary or combined therapy. It is unclear if garlic reduces postmeal blood sugar levels or hemoglobin A_{1c} levels.

SUMMARY

Garlic is a plant that has been a necessity in everyday life from the past until the present day. Today, garlic as well as garlic preparations is prescribed in many pharmacopoeias in the world; it contains active compounds that are responsible for its effect on almost every part of the human body. It has been used for a plethora of medical conditions from ancient times to current day treatments. Evidence supports that the administration of garlic should not be avoided; on the contrary, its intake should be as much as possible because it underlies human health.

CLINICS CARE POINTS

- Garlic has shown to be effective in the treatment of numerous disease processes.

- Garlic is inexpensive, antibacterial and has been used since ancient times to the present.
- Garlic is most effective when used with traditional Western medicinal modalities.

DISCLOSURE

The author has nothing to disclose.

REFERENCES

1. "Garlic." Merriam-Webster.com Dictionary, Merriam-Webster. Available at: https://www.merriam-webster.com/dictionary/garlic. Accessed July 9, 2020.
2. Cambridge Dictionary Cambridge University press 2020 Online. Available at: https://dictionary.cambridge.org/. Accessed January 18, 2021.
3. Bauer Petrovska B, Cekovska S. Extracts from the history and medical properties of garlic. Pharmacogn Rev 2010;4(7):106–10.
4. Tweed V. Put more garlic in your life (magzter.com). Available at: https://www.magzter.com/stories/Health/Better-Nutrition/Put-More-Garlic-In-Your-Life. Accessed January 18, 2021.
5. Hirst K, Kris. Garlic domestication - where did it come from and when?. 2020. Available at: https://www.thoughtco.com/garlic-domestication-where-and-when-169374 Images News/Getty Images. Accessed January 18, 2021.
6. Vegetariantimes.com APRIL 2016 pg 22 – 24 In Praise of Garlc by Karen Asp.
7. Bayan L, Koulivand PH, Gorji A. Garlic: a review of potential therapeutic effects. Avicenna J Phytomed 2014;4(1):1–14.
8. Yang C, Li L, Yang L, et al. Anti-obesity and hypolipidemic effects of garlic oil and onion oil in rats fed a high-fat diet. Nutr Metab 2018;15(1):43.
9. Berry C. Natural alternatives for infection. Nutritional perspectives. J Counc Nutr 2018;41(4):12–3. Available at: https://search-ebscohost-com.ezproxy.lib.apsu.edu/login.aspx?direct=true&db=ccm&AN=142103616&site=ehost-live&scope=site. Accessed July 7, 2020.
10. Lissiman E, Bhasale AL, Cohen M. Garlic for the common cold. Cochrane Database Syst Rev 2014;Issue 11:cd006206. Rodrigo A, Sarar Quintero-Fabian.
11. Arreola R, Quintero-Fabián S, López-Roa RI, et al. Immunomodulation and anti-inflammatory effects of garlic compounds. J Immunol Res 2015;2015:401630.

Printed and bound by CPI Group (UK) Ltd, Croydon, CR0 4YY

03/10/2024

01040407-0012